Remediation of /r/
for
Speech-Language
Pathologists

Remediation of /r/
for
Speech-Language Pathologists

Peter Flipsen Jr., PhD, S-LP(C), CCC-SLP

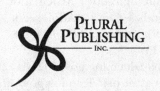

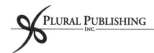

5521 Ruffin Road
San Diego, CA 92123

e-mail: information@pluralpublishing.com
Website: https://www.pluralpublishing.com

Typeset in 11/13 Garamond by Flanagan's Publishing Services, Inc.
Printed in the United States of America by McNaughton & Gunn, Inc.

Library of Congress Cataloging-in-Publication Data:

Names: Flipsen, Peter, Jr., author.
Title: Remediation of /r/ for speech-language pathologists / Peter Flipsen
  Jr.
Description: San Diego, CA : Plural Publishing, Inc., [2022] | Includes
  bibliographical references and index.
Identifiers: LCCN 2021011287 (print) | LCCN 2021011288 (ebook) | ISBN
  9781635502879 (paperback) | ISBN 9781635503029 (ebook)
Subjects: MESH: Speech Intelligibility | Articulation Disorders—therapy |
  Speech Therapy—methods | Child | Adolescent
Classification: LCC RJ496.S7 (print) | LCC RJ496.S7 (ebook) | NLM WV 501
  | DDC 618.92/855—dc23
LC record available at https://lccn.loc.gov/2021011287
LC ebook record available at https://lccn.loc.gov/2021011288

Contents

Preface: A Visit With the Rhotacist   vii
Reviewers   xi

Chapter 1. Introduction   1

Chapter 2. Typical Production of American English /r/   19

Chapter 3. When to Intervene   33

Chapter 4. Assessment of /r/   43

Chapter 5. Remediation Principles   73

Chapter 6. Treatment Option 1: Fine-Tuning Traditional   101
Articulation Therapy

Chapter 7. Treatment Option 2: Modifying Traditional   129
Articulation Therapy

Chapter 8. Treatment Option 3: Adding Supplemental   143
Tactile Feedback

Chapter 9. Treatment Option 4: Adding Visual Feedback   155
via Electropalatography

Chapter 10. Treatment Option 5: Adding Visual Acoustic   169
Feedback

Chapter 11. Treatment Option 6: Adding Visual Feedback   185
via Ultrasound

Chapter 12. Concluding Remarks: Deciding What to Do   197

References   201
Index   219

Preface

A Visit With the Rhotacist

In my more than 20 years of teaching in speech pathology programs and presenting at various professional meetings, I hear a lot about problems with remediating /r/ errors, especially with children over age 8 years. I am quite regularly approached by clinicians, including those with a wide range of clinical experience, who vent their frustration with this target sound. The most common query is "got any tricks?" I readily sympathize. I still recall my own challenges dealing with these errors in my clinical practice back in Canada in the early 1990s. It is also not uncommon for current students in their clinic placements to approach me after class for help correcting an aberrant /r/, often noting that they and their supervisors have "run out of ideas." Although I cannot promise any quick fixes here, I hope this book will at least offer some direction.

Specific concern about /r/ is not a new phenomenon. At least as early as 1882, Samuel Potter referred to this sound as "the most difficult consonant" (p. 34). He also referred to errors on /r/ as *rhotacism*. The word is derived from "rhotic" that is a label typically attached to /r/. Although the label rhotacism has long been out of favor, it was briefly revived a century later by Shriberg[1] (1982). In a book chapter discussing a very different kind of speech problem, Shriberg made reference to the *rhotacist2* or specialist in the correction of /r/ errors. Although I hesitate to consider myself such a specialist, for purposes of this book, I will attempt to serve as your friendly neighborhood rhotacist.

Rather than calling it rhoticism, most clinicians these days just describe the specific error being produced. For example, they may mention a "distortion of /r/" or a "substitution of [w] for /r/." The latter type of error (an overt substitution) is more common in preschool children; such substitutions rarely persist past age 6 years and either resolve into fully correct /r/

---

[1]In the interests of full disclosure, Shriberg was my doctoral mentor. His early research focused on the treatment of /r/; thus, this book is somewhat of a homage to him.

[2]Shriberg actually attributes the term to John Locke (a researcher in speech pathology, not the 17th-century philosopher).

or transform slightly into the other type of error (a distortion), which is intermediate between /w/ and /r/. These distortions are what we usually observe in children older than age 7 years and in adults. Although our main focus here is on those older children and those distortions, most of the approaches for remediating /r/ errors to be discussed herein will apply to other groups and to [w] for /r/ substitutions.

Most children with /r/ errors ultimately end up with fully normal speech. Many do so on their own, while others do so following intervention with our current approaches. Unfortunately, not all of them do. Although the specific proportion of children who fail to do so is not known, the level of interest by clinicians suggests that the numbers are not trivial. For example, at the 2013 convention of the American Speech-Language-Hearing Association (ASHA) in Chicago, Illinois, I copresented a seminar on an approach that has been applied to remediating /r/ (Sacks & Flipsen, 2013) that is discussed in Chapter 7. The room, which had a capacity of about 200, was filled to overflowing, and it was necessary to also broadcast it to another room. On another occasion, I was specifically asked to address this challenge for a 2014 workshop that I gave for about 30 speech-language pathologists in the Beaverton (Oregon) School District. A 2015 special issue of the journal *Seminars in Speech and Language* was also devoted to the topic. Finally, at my presentation for the 2018 Oregon Speech and Hearing Association's spring rural conference, most of the questions I fielded from the over 100 attendees related to dealing with persistent speech errors (especially /r/) in older children.

Given the frequency of the questions, it has become clear to me that current approaches are not universally effective. What I mean here by current approaches is traditional articulation therapy. According to Brumbaugh and Smit (2013) this is what most clinicians do, and admittedly, it is what I tell my students to at least start with. The questions also suggest that most clinicians either appear to assume that is all they can do, or even if they are aware of alternatives, are not certain where to start.

Thankfully, there are alternatives available with evidence to support their effectiveness. Some of these approaches have actually been around for a long time (e.g., electropalatography and spectrograms), while others (e.g., ultrasound) have emerged only recently. Despite what many clinicians believe, several of them are well within the practical reach of most, including those who work in the public schools. Still others are not yet practical for school-based application (mostly from a cost perspective), but they deserve mention here as those in medical and/or private practice settings may well be able to justify the costs involved. Having collected information on these approaches (and contributed to the development of at least one of them) for several years now and shared them with my own students, I have felt for some time that clinicians needed a source that brought together information on these methods—hence, this book.

The target reading audience for what is contained herein is primarily practicing clinicians (i.e., speech-language pathologists) and/or advanced graduate students in the field. Thus, I will assume some basic knowledge of phonetics, acoustics, and the basic elements of speech remediation.

The goal here is to offer practicing clinicians the most up-to-date information on what we know about /r/, the errors related to /r/, and the range of approaches available for their remediation. It also includes a detailed review and evaluation of the existing literature and a discussion of current approaches. I will say from the outset that *at least some* of our challenge with /r/ may be that we are not being systematic enough. Our recent learnings about "principles of motor learning," for example, are not yet as widely applied as they should be. As well, there are ways to reorganize or tweak traditional articulation therapy that have been shown to make it more effective. The Challenge Point Framework, to be discussed, offers one way for us to do so. There are others. Chapter 6 in fact is devoted to fine-tuning traditional therapy.

That said, even with fine-tuning, traditional articulation therapy may not work in all cases. Other approaches may be needed. This book also includes a discussion of several very promising alternative treatment approaches that do not yet seem to have made it onto the radar of most practicing clinicians (or if they have it is not clear to many whether they are viable for most clinicians to implement). The idea is to present these approaches in a way consistent with evidence-based practice (EBP; ASHA, 2005) by discussing the emerging evidence along with at least some guidance about implementing them. I hope to be able to do so in a way that is inherently practical (i.e., with enough detail so that they can be applied). I also strongly encourage the reader to go to the primary sources I cite for additional information.

Readers may notice that a few approaches have not been included. There are two reasons for this. First, only approaches where empirical evidence that has undergone some level of peer review are included. That means some data supporting their use have been either published in a journal or presented at a professional conference. I apologize in advance if something has been missed. Second, there are at least three approaches where, although they theoretically could be applied to children with /r/ errors, the only available evidence for them is for individuals with much more severe involvement. These include top-down approaches like *Whole-Language Intervention* (Hoffman & Norris, 2010) or *Naturalistic Intervention* (Camarata, 2021). Both of these might logically have been included in Chapter 7 because they involve ignoring the traditional therapy progression by working exclusively at the conversational speech level. However, neither of these were included here primarily because they both involve feedback that tends to be about whether the message was actually understood or not. However, the speech of older children with only one or two errors is typically quite easy to understand. Applying these approaches would require a lot of pretending to misunderstand on the part of the clinician. This might be a challenge to maintain for very long. The third approach that readers might wonder about is PROMPT© (Hayden et al., 2021), which might logically have been included in Chapter 8. Much of its focus is on supplemental tactile feedback. Although there is some evidence supporting its use, the evidence is focused on individuals with much more severe involvement. Indeed, it tends to be presented as intended for such individuals. I was unable to identify any empirical evidence specifically supporting its use with older children with only a few errors. That is not to say that it could not successfully be applied to such clients. We simply cannot know one way or the other whether it would work.

Before diving into the heart of the matter, I should thank a few people. First, I need to thank my current and former colleagues in the School of Communication Sciences and Disorders at Pacific University for encouraging me in this endeavor. They have, each in their own way, helped make this happen. In particular, several have regularly asked for or commented about an outline for this book that has been displayed on the whiteboard in my office for several years. Thanks also to Elaine Hitchcock, Tara McAllister, Gordy Rogers, Jonathan Preston, Stephen Sacks, and Steven Skelton for vital comments and input on specific elements of the book. Special thanks to Amy Neel for generating the LPC images for Chapter 10 and to the following for providing other images: Stephen Sacks (Chapter 6), Abigail Anderson (Chapter 8), Christian Chidester (Chapter 9), Paul Sharp (Chapter 9), Jonathon Preston (Chapter 11), and Jane Timmis (Chapter 11). I am especially indebted to Angie Singh and her staff at Plural Publishing (in particular, my editor Christina Gunning) for their willingness to work with me to bring this book to fruition. Of course, many thanks to my wife Patricia for her support and patience throughout this process.

Finally, I must make my disclosures. I have no financial relationships or interests to disclose that might represent a conflict of interest. In the spirit of openness, I must mention something relative to the SATPAC approach to be discussed primarily in Chapter 7. I have assisted the developer of that program (Stephen Sacks) with designing studies to test his approach and with disseminating the results. I do not, however, receive anything (financial or otherwise) from him or his company for doing so. I should also note that I am employed as a full-time, tenured professor by Pacific University, Oregon, and was given a one-semester (Spring 2020) sabbatical leave to write this book. It counts toward my expected scholarship, but (consistent with academic freedom) I appreciate that I was not restricted in any way about what I wrote. I do not have any nonfinancial relationships or interests to disclose.

Reviewers

Plural Publishing and the author would like to thank the following reviewers for taking the time to provide their valuable feedback during the manuscript development process. Additional anonymous feedback was provided by other expert reviewers.

Kay Alley, MS, CCC-SLP
Speech-Language Pathologist
Roanoke City Public Schools
Roanoke, Virginia

Julie Beard, PhD, CCC-SLP
Assistant Professor
Auburn University at Montgomery
Montgomery, Alabama

Jennifer Binkley, MS, CCC-SLP
Instructor
Abilene Christian University
Abilene, Texas

Lauren E. Bland, PhD, CCC-SLP
Associate Professor/Graduate
 Program Director
Western Kentucky University
Bowling Green, Kentucky

**Alycia Cummings, PhD,
CCC-SLP**
Associate Professor
Idaho State University
Pocatello, Idaho

Carol M. Ellis, PhD, CCC-SLP
Associate Professor
Fort Hays State University
Hays, Kansas

David Eoute, Jr., PhD, CCC-SLP
Associate Professor
Bob Jones University
Greenville, South Carolina

**Jennifer Glassman, PhD,
CCC-SLP CHES**
Assistant Professor
University of Toledo
Toledo, Ohio

Leisa Harmon, MS, CCC-SLP
Assistant Professor
Minot State University
Minot, North Dakota

Robert McKinney, MA, CCC-SLP
Speech-Language Pathologist
Sweetwater Union High School
 District
Chula Vista, California

Megan S. Overby, PhD, CCC-SLP
Associate Professor
Duquesne University
Pittsburgh, Pennsylvania

Samantha Pannone, MA, CCC-SLP
Speech-Language Pathologist
Silver Spring, Maryland

Lucia Pasquel-Lefebvre, MA, CCC-SLP
Speech-Language Pathologist/
   Owner
Holistic Kids, PLLC
Durham, North Carolina

Suzanne Podberesky, MA, CCC-SLP
Speech-Language Pathologist
Montgomery County Public Schools
Rockville, Maryland

Debra Schober-Peterson, PhD, CCC-SLP, BCS-CL
Clinical Professor, Director of
   Clinical Education
Georgia State University
Atlanta, Georgia

Amy L. Vaughn, PhD, CCC-SLP
Assistant Professor
Baldwin Wallace University
Berea, Ohio

CHAPTER 1

Introduction

This chapter lays the groundwork for much of the rest of the book. It discusses the scope of the problem, the particular clinical challenges posed by /r/, and whether working on these errors can be justified. It includes an overview of the methods being used to study /r/ and other speech sounds and establishes a framework for symbols to be used to represent /r/. It also includes a brief discussion of evidence-based practice.

SCOPE OF THE PROBLEM

Approximately 10% of preschool children[1] have at least some difficulty with the production of speech sounds (Bernthal et al., 2017). Relative to typical caseloads (i.e., those we actually serve), a study of 597 clinicians supporting almost 15,000 students from 37 states indicated that about 75% of pre-K caseloads involve working on speech sounds at least some of the time. That number drops to about 56% in K–3 caseloads and drops further to about 22% in caseloads for Grades 7 through 12 (Mullen & Schooling, 2010). Thus, even by the time they reach high school, up to one fifth of the children we serve still require work on speech sounds. Unfortunately, even in high school, we do not seem to be solving all of these problems. This is seen in the fact that 1% to 2% of adults retain mild (typically distortion)

---

[1]The terms *child*, *client*, *speaker*, *patient*, and *student* will be used somewhat interchangeably throughout this book to reflect the variety of terms used and the variety of settings in which speech-language pathologists (SLPs) work.

errors on /s/ or /r/[2] in their speech (Flipsen, 2015). If this were baseball, we would probably be ecstatic. A trend going from 10% of preschoolers down to 1% to 2% of adults suggests we have a success rate of 80% to 90%. In baseball that would be an incredible batting average, but alas, this is not a game. A failure to successfully treat 10% to 20% of our patients is nothing to crow about, particularly when speech sound intervention is supposed to be so central to what we do. This failure rate is not only high, but it is also common across clinicians; a survey of 200 clinicians by Ruscello (1995a) suggested that 91% have worked with clients who failed to master one or more speech sounds.

Adults with persistent and residual errors (we discuss the difference between those terms in Chapter 3) are producing errors on either /s/ or /r/ or both. Our focus here is on /r/. While there is no good empirical evidence on the proportion of cases that specifically involve /r/, if the relative frequency of questions raised by clinicians is any indication, it appears that /r/ represents a significant portion of the load. We might also infer this from the fact that we see more males than females with speech sound disorders overall, and /r/ errors are more common in males[3] (see Shriberg, 2010).

THE PARTICULAR CHALLENGE OF /r/

What is it about /r/ that makes it such a challenge for us to remediate? Why is it that /r/ remains for us what Potter (1882) called, "the most difficult consonant" (p. 34)? Our challenges with correcting or remediating aberrant productions appear to be the result of many interacting factors. Not all of these factors apply in each case, but at least some of them are likely to apply to many of them. For convenience, I grouped these factors into those related to /r/ itself, those related to us as clinicians, and those related to the therapy process. Addressing many of these factors to improve what we are doing is the focus of much of the rest of this book.

Target-Related Factors

1. *An /r/ does not involve very much physical contact between the tongue and the rest of the vocal tract.* This is why many texts refer to /r/

---

[2]For the sake of brevity, unless discussed separately, the symbol /r/ will be assumed to include both consonant and vocalic forms of this sound (this distinction is discussed later). This usage is also consistent with that of Ladefoged (2005).

[3]It is worth noting that /s/ errors are more common in females (Shriberg, 2010).

as an "approximant." It only involves a general narrowing of the vocal tract (i.e., it approximates a constriction). The net result is that speakers receive only minimal tactile feedback from the vocal tract to use both while learning to produce the sound and when self-monitoring their ongoing productions.

2. */r/ requires controlled constriction at three different points in the vocal tract during its production (lips, palate, pharynx).* Most other speech sounds require only a single point of constriction, or at most, two points. Thus, /r/ involves much more articulatory coordination than is required for most other speech sounds. It also requires controlling two different parts of the tongue in different ways at the same time. It has been argued (Gick et al., 2007) that the common substitution pattern ([w] for /r/) reflects an attempt to replace those two independent movements with a single one (i.e., simply moving the dorsum of the tongue toward the velum rather than adjusting the root of the tongue for a pharyngeal constriction and simultaneously adjusting the dorsum of the tongue for an oral constriction).

3. *There are multiple ways to produce a fully correct /r/.* Several investigators (e.g., Delattre & Freeman, 1968; Hagiwara, 1995; Westbury et al., 1998) have shown that typical speakers can use a variety of tongue shapes and still yield the same perceptually correct /r/.

Clinician-Related Factors[4]

1. *A fixation with a retroflex tongue shape.* There has been a long-standing assumption among many clinicians that a retroflex (tongue curling back on itself) shape is the only way to produce a good /r/.[5] Although good data are lacking, at least one other possibility, a "bunched" tongue shape, may actually be used at least as often as a retroflex shape.

2. *The constraints of categorical perception.* Our natural tendency, as competent users of the language, is to want to put the speaker's production into a specific phonemic category in the language. In the case of American English /r/, when judging their productions,

---

[4]My apologies if these come across as "blaming the clinician"; that is certainly not the intent. However, we need to acknowledge that sometimes our failure to solve the patient's problem may, at least in part, reflect our own inadequate knowledge or skills. The fact that you are reading this book suggests you want to change that. I applaud your desire to serve your patients better.

[5]There appears to be a trend away from this assumption among more recently trained clinicians.

we want to call it either /r/ or /w/. Unfortunately, many of those we serve (particularly those above age 7 years) produce a version that is neither. As a resonant sound, speakers are capable of producing many versions of /r/ that are intermediate between /r/ and /w/. In the case of productions that are not clearly either of those (i.e., that are distortions), many of us struggle with what feedback to provide. Sometimes we have difficulty discerning the difference. Even when we recognize that it is not fully correct, do we call it correct? Do we call it incorrect? Perhaps more importantly, are we being consistent in our judgments and the feedback we provide?

3. *Ignoring speech perception.* This is a challenge for much of speech sound intervention. We tend to want to jump right into production training. While it is true that general problems of speech perception are rarely an issue for children with speech sound disorders, *some errors by some children* may reflect an underlying perceptual problem. That means they may have difficulty hearing the difference between what they say and what they are supposed to say for that specific sound. It is possible that some of the /r/ errors we are treating as production errors may need to also be treated as problems based in perception.

4. *Ignoring the pharyngeal constriction.* The feedback we provide to our patients regarding how to change their productions has focused almost exclusively on what to do with the body and front portion of the tongue (with an occasional mention of the lips). It rarely involves doing anything with the tongue root or the pharynx. In fairness, until recently, studies of normal /r/ production have largely ignored the pharynx, so we know little about what should be happening there. Even if we did, none of us really knows what sort of feedback to provide in that area to help our patients change what they are doing. Ignoring it may, however be a critical issue for some clients.

Therapy-Related Factors

1. *The Challenge of Bad Habits.* Although not a problem that is limited to /r/, by the time most clinicians begin working on this sound at age 7 to 8 years of age, our clients have had many years of practicing their errors. Given what are often brief therapy sessions, they have a lot of other time where they are continuing to practice those errors. Since most of these distortion errors do not interfere with intelligibility, they are also effectively being reinforced (or at least not being penalized) by the rest of the world. The result is a highly ingrained habit, which can be difficult to break.

2. *Demographic Dynamics.* This one involves some speculation on my part. When we provide models for our patient to imitate in therapy, one view is that the patient tries to create in the mind (on some level) an internal image of the clinician's vocal tract shape. The client then tries to re-create that specific vocal tract shape when attempting to imitate the sound. This idea arises from what has been called the *motor theory of speech perception.* As mentioned earlier, more of our /r/ patients will be males, but most clinicians are female. As discussed in Chapter 2 (and as you may have learned in your phonetics or anatomy classes as an undergraduate student), male and female vocal tracts are organized slightly differently. The lengths of the oral cavity and the pharyngeal cavity are approximately equal in females, but (in relative terms) the oral cavity is shorter than the pharyngeal cavity in males. Hagiwara (1995) has suggested that this means that males and females have to create both the oral and pharyngeal constrictions for /r/ at relatively different locations in order to achieve the same acoustic output. It is therefore possible that some male patients may struggle to reproduce a good /r/ if their only models in therapy are from females. The model they are hearing reflects a vocal tract that is organized differently than the one they are using to try to generate the sound. At the very least, it suggests that if we have a patient whose problem with /r/ is partly one of perception, it may be crucial to provide a variety of different speaker models (i.e., including both males and females) to improve both perception and production.

SHOULD WE WORRY ABOUT /r/ ERRORS IN OLDER CHILDREN?

Given the title of this book, this question is obviously rhetorical. It is however worth asking, because some clinicians and some academics in the field have questioned whether intervention for these errors is actually justified. While some of this may reflect frustration with our lack of success with some of our patients and be simply a search for reasons to walk away, there are defendable reasons for not working on these sounds. For example, when we are talking about distortion errors produced by older children and adults, comprehension by listeners is rarely an issue—almost everyone is able to understand the intended message. This may actually be the main reason many of these errors persist. There is usually little motivation to change anything when it is getting the job done.

A second reason for not working on these errors is that unlike the substitution errors seen in younger children that have been shown to impact reading and writing skills, in the past it has been assumed that distortion errors do not impact these skills. Although recent literature has suggested that may not be the case, if that is the assumption, then we might ask: What problem are we solving?

A third argument against being concerned about these errors draws from the diversity perspective. Distortions of /r/ are actually a normal part of the speech pattern of some major American dialects (e.g., Southern English, Bostonian English, Appalachian English), although in those dialects the changes tend to be limited only to /r/ sounds in postvocalic (i.e., final) position. The same is true for several non-American varieties of English (e.g., British English, Australian English, New Zealand English). Could we not simply assume that these distortion errors represent a "difference" rather than a "disorder"?

Finally, there are data to suggest (see Flipsen, 2015) that up to 75% of these errors resolve on their own (i.e., without intervention) between about age 9 years and the end of high school.

Despite such justifications, most clinicians take the view that these errors are worth correcting (or at least attempting to do so). They argue that it is not at all clear how to separate those children whose errors will resolve on their own from those whose errors will not do so. Perhaps more importantly, there can be significant negative impacts of these errors on both immediate and long-term quality of life. For example, an Australian study of over four thousand 7- to 9-year-olds (McCormack et al., 2011) reported that compared to those without communication impairments, significantly more bullying was experienced by those with communication impairments. Crowe Hall (1991) reported that fourth and sixth graders with mild speech errors (both /s/ and /r/) were viewed significantly more negatively by their peers. Silverman and Paulus (1989) reported similar findings for high school sophomores who produced /r/ errors. Finally, individuals with even these mild distortion errors may also be less likely to be hired (see Cronin et al., 2014), especially for jobs that involve significant interaction with the public. Individuals who produce these errors may therefore face more limited career prospects.

Farquharson (2019) has provided additional rationale for working on single sound errors. She argues against the idea that single sound errors do not impact reading. Many (but not all) of these children have had histories of multiple speech errors and have spent prolonged periods in therapy. Having mastered much of their speech sound system later than their peers, they may have failed to make crucial associations between spoken and written language. Perhaps more importantly, their underlying representations for any remaining production errors such as /r/ may be poorly developed; this may make it difficult for them to make a consistent association between the sound and its spelling equivalents. This would not be trivial for /r/, which is one of the more common sounds in the English language (see Mines et al., 1978).

CAN WE JUSTIFY WORKING ON /r/ ERRORS IN OLDER CHILDREN?

Despite taking the philosophical position that we should work on these errors, many clinicians who work in U.S. public schools face a potential bureaucratic hurdle. Many have been told by their supervisors or other clinicians that a child who only presents with one or two speech errors does not qualify for services under federal law if they are performing adequately in academic subjects. They point to the regulations for implementing the U.S. Individuals with Disabilities Education Act (IDEA, 2004) that state that the disability must "adversely affect educational performance." A survey by Farquharson and Boldini (2018) found a great deal of variability in how school-based clinicians interpret this concept. Many assume that "educational performance" is the same as academic achievement, and if the speech issue cannot be linked to failure in academic subjects, the child is not eligible to receive services for speech.

However, the idea that a child must be failing academically in order to qualify for speech services appears to be a misinterpretation of the federal regulations. In 2006, the American Speech-Language-Hearing Association (ASHA) sought guidance from the federal government on this question. The response came in a letter dated March 8, 2007, from Alexa Posny, Director of the U.S. Office of Special Education Programs. Ms. Posny stated the following:

> It remains the Department's position that the term "educational performance" as used in the IDEA and its implementing regulations is not limited to academic performance. Whether a speech and language impairment adversely affects a child's educational performance must be determined on a case-by-case basis, depending on the unique needs of a particular child and *not based only on discrepancies in age or grade performance in academic subject areas* [emphasis added]. (Office of Special Education and Rehabilitative Services, 2007, para. 2)

This suggests that a child does *not* need to be underperforming academically in order to qualify for speech services. The negative social, communication, or other nonacademic impacts of a speech problem should be, by themselves, sufficient to qualify a child for services under federal law. This notion is supported by a Campbell Law Review article by Thomas (2016) who notes that educational is not the same as academic, specifically stating the following:

> The plain meaning of the word "educational" seems to reference not only academic learning but also social, emotional, and interpersonal

development. The theme underlying both the definitions and the etymological origins is one of equipping an individual with a variety of skills and preparing him/her for "mature" or independent life. (p. 86)

> **Box 1–1**
>
> Academic failure is not necessary to qualify a child for services to remediate speech sound errors in the U.S. public schools.

It is worth noting that parents of children with /r/ errors appear to agree that academic performance need not be the primary motivator for working to remediate such errors. A survey of the parents of 91 of these children reported greater concern with the negative social impacts of their child's speech than with how they might affect academics (Hitchcock et al., 2015).

APPROACHES TO STUDYING /r/

In order to better understand our recent learnings about /r/ and to orient us to some of the new approaches for remediating /r/ errors, it seems appropriate to offer a bit of a primer/refresher regarding the different approaches to understanding speech production in general and /r/ in particular. Several of these are also now the basis for some of the alternative approaches to be discussed in later chapters.

Early efforts to understand speech involved simply looking inside speakers' mouths to see and/or asking them to describe what was happening. Early speech scientists would also try to describe what they felt was happening inside their own mouths. This approach has obvious limitations. Most of us have little conscious awareness of what is happening in our vocal tracts. Also, much of what is happening inside the mouth during speech is not easily visible (even with the aid of flashlights) either because opening the mouth to get a good view changes the configuration being used or our vision of the back of the oral cavity or pharynx is blocked by the tongue. These limitations have motivated the development of several technologies to help us understand what is happening inside the vocal tract.

Palatography

One of the first technologies to be developed to assist with understanding speech is called *palatography.* This involves documenting the pattern of contact between the tongue and the palate during speech. In its earliest forms, this involved painting ink or dye onto a speaker's palate, having them produce a single speech sound, and then taking a photograph (either directly or using a mirror) of the palate. The areas where the dye was no longer present were the places where the tongue had made contact. This approach was used as early as the 1870s (see Fletcher, 1992, for a discussion). It had very limited usefulness, however, in that only a single sound produced by itself could be examined; as such it is sometimes called *static palatography*.

In the 1950s, the notion of an artificial palate was introduced (see Ladefoged, 1957), which involved taking an impression of the speaker's upper teeth and palate. This was then used to create an acrylic device that could be covered in dye, inserted into the speaker's mouth, and then removed after the speaker produced a sound or a word. Again, the pattern of tongue to palate could be viewed.

In the 1960s, researchers such as Samuel Fletcher and others expanded on the notion of an artificial palate by developing what they called *dynamic palatometry*; this has more recently been referred to as *electropalatography* (EPG). The artificial palate or *pseudopalate* would be embedded with multiple tiny sensors that could detect the pressure of contact from the tongue. Each sensor is connected to a tiny wire, and all these wires are bundled together and hang out of the mouth. The wires are then connected to a computer screen that can display the pattern of tongue to palate contact. Figure 1–1 illustrates the functional elements of this approach. The rightmost image is the cast used to create the pseudopalate (shown in the middle image). The small black dots throughout the pseudopalate represent the pressure sensors, and there are some horizontal wires on each side that clip onto the teeth to hold the pseudopalate in place. The leftmost image in Figure 1–1 is an example of a display showing the pattern of tongue-to-palate contact (the front of the mouth is at the top); in this case, it shows a static production of a normal /s/. The dark squares are the points of contact, and the clear squares are points of no contact. As might be expected, tongue contact can be seen all along the right and left sides. This reflects the sides of the tongue sealing off the teeth for /s/. The result is that air is forced down the narrow channel created in the center of the tongue where airflow for a normal /s/ is directed. The lack of contact (the clear square) near the center of Row 1 is the opening just behind the upper central incisors where air escapes to generate the characteristic hissing sound of /s/.

The newer version of this approach is called dynamic palatography because, in principle, a consecutive set of images could be taken while speech is ongoing to see how contact between tongue and palate changes over time across words or phrases. Until recently, the limitations of computer power made such dynamic imaging impractical, but recent computer advances now allow for many images per second to be generated and stored. Software is now either cloud based or runs on most laptops.

Row	EPG frame of the maximum point of contact for /s/	Region of palate	Hypothesized area of tongue	EPG palate	Dental cast with junction between hard and soft palate drawn
1 2 3 4 5 6 7 8	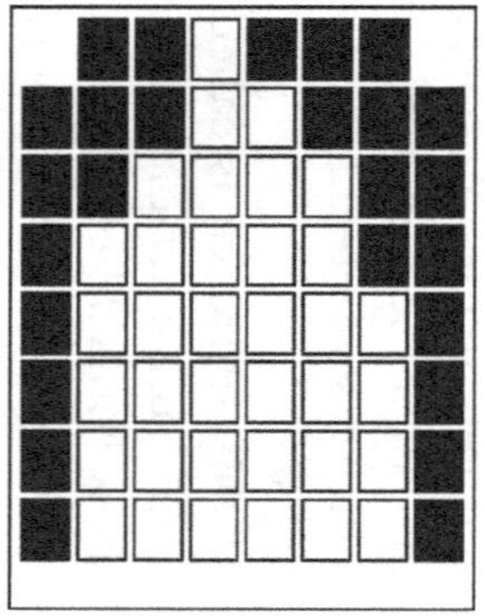	Alveolar (2 rows) Palatal (3 rows) Velar (3 rows)	Anterior (tip) Blade Posterior (body)	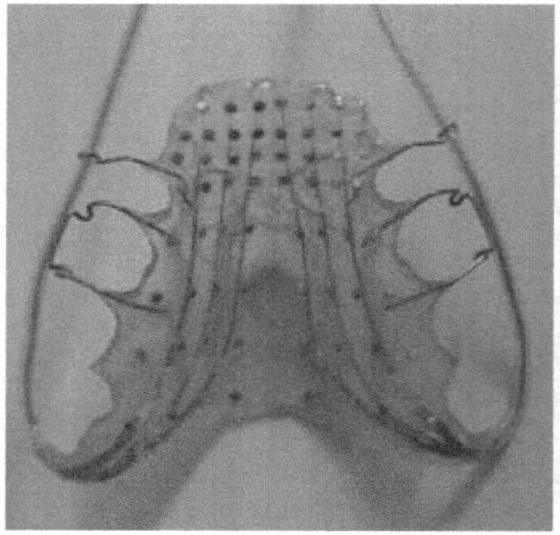	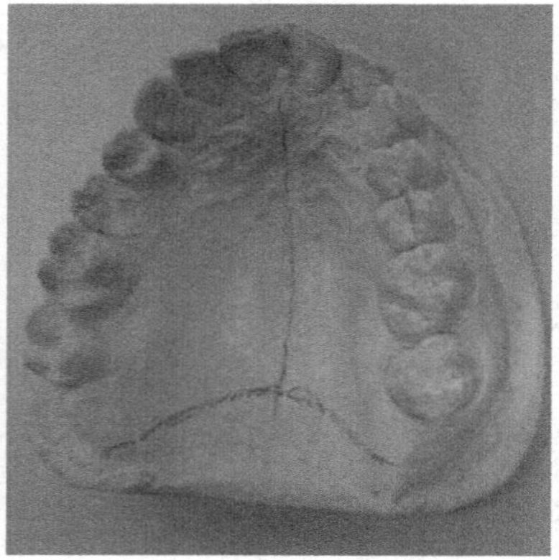

Figure 1–1. Functional elements of electropalatograpy. From *Seeing Speech: A Quick Guide to Speech Sounds* by Sharynne McLeod and Sadanand Singh, 2009. p. xi. Copyright 2009 by Plural Publishing. All Rights Reserved.

Another previous limitation of EPG, which prevented its widespread use for research or clinical application, was the fact that pseudopalates might cost several thousands of dollars each to construct. Given the unique nature of each person's palate shape and size, they are also only usable by a single speaker. In recent years, the cost of creating pseudopalates has decreased considerably, though they are still on the order of several hundred dollars each. The net result of these recent developments is that EPG for remediation of speech sound errors has seen a significant increase in use in both research and clinical application. Although it may not yet be viable for use in the public schools, it is now being used by some in private practice. Its use for remediating /r/ is discussed in Chapter 9.

X-Rays

Another indirect method for studying speech emerged with the development of x-ray imaging in the early part of the 20th century. Many of the midsagittal images shown in our phonetics textbooks were originally made by tracing tongue shapes in x-ray images. Serious concerns about the health risks of exposure to ionizing radiation, however, have limited the application of this technology. A few descriptive studies have been carried out (e.g., Kuehn & Tomblin, 1977).

In the 1980s and 1990s, a short-lived approach attempted to use the power of x-rays in a way that would both reduce x-ray risks and capture the growing power of computers. It was called the *x-ray microbeam* and involved the creation of a multi-million-dollar device (of which only two were ever built) that stretched the length of about two large public school classrooms. At one end, the "subject" was seated in a small booth with a series of tiny gold pellets glued to the center of their tongue and on several other anatomical landmarks (cervical spine, mandible, upper lip). The speaker was then asked to produce a variety of utterances, and a tiny beam of x-rays was directed at the gold pellets, while a then-quite-powerful computer tracked their movements. The net result was supposed to be the ability to study speech production in a very dynamic way with minimal x-ray exposure. Despite their promise, only a limited amount of research was ever published using the data from these devices, and they have since both been decommissioned. It also appears that no child data were ever collected. However, we can learn some things from the available evidence, and we discuss some of it in Chapter 2.

Ultrasound

The need to use gold pellets in the x-ray microbeam highlights one of the very real limitations of x-rays, namely, that they do not provide very detailed images of soft tissue such as the tongue and velum (though they do very well with dense material such as bone or gold pellets). To make up for that limitation, another technology was developed that has been widely used in medicine for a few decades. It is ultrasound, in which high-frequency sound waves are passed through various body tissues, and patterns of reflectance are measured to yield images of the structures.[6] Although initially an extremely expensive technology, the cost has come down considerably in recent years, making it a viable technique for researching speech production. Studies using ultrasound to study speech and speech remediation have proliferated in the last 15 years or so. Although still too expensive for most clinical use, it is starting to be used in a few private practice settings. An example of an ultrasound image that shows the tongue at rest is in Figure 1–2. This particular image is a midsagittal view with the speaker facing to the right. The bright white (mostly horizontal) line running across the middle of the image is the hard palate, and the tongue is visible as the slightly less bright mass immediately

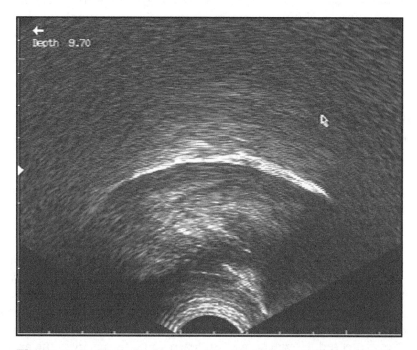

Figure 1–2. Ultrasound image of the tongue at rest. Midsagittal view with speaker facing to the right. From *Seeing Speech: A Quick Guide to Speech Sounds* by Sharynne McLeod and Sadanand Singh, 2009, p, x. Copyright 2009 Plural Publishing. All Rights Reserved.

---

[6]Ultrasound actually does poorly at providing fine detail of the palate, jaw, and hyoid bone because sound waves are refracted off their hard, curved surfaces (see Stone, 1990).

below the center of that. The application of ultrasound to remediation of /r/ errors is discussed in Chapter 11.

Acoustic Analysis

Speech can be described as either the patterns of shapes and movements created by the articulators within the vocal tract or the resulting patterns of vibrations in the air that reach a listener's ear. Acoustic analysis involves analysis of those vibrations. The first formal treatise on displaying visual patterns that represent speech output appears to have been the 1947 book *Visible Speech* by Potter, Kopp, and Green. Much research on normal speech production has been carried out with this technology. Over the years, these analyses have also been shown to be useful for providing visual feedback for remediating errors on speech sounds such as /r/ (e.g., Shuster et al., 1995).

Although most clinicians learned about the power of this tool in their training programs at some point, most continue to assume that it is both too expensive and too cumbersome for clinical application. Although true of early versions of this technology, neither is true any longer. Acoustic analysis software is now available (mostly free) and will operate on the laptop computers that most clinicians already use in their daily clinical practice. The only necessary addition might be a relatively inexpensive external microphone.

Several types of acoustic analysis displays are possible that have been shown to have clinical usefulness (e.g., Ertmer & Maki, 2000; Shuster et al., 1992). For example, spectrogram displays show frequency by time, waveform displays show amplitude by time, and linear predictive coding (LPC) spectral displays show amplitude by frequency. The application of this tool is discussed in more detail in Chapter 10.

Other Approaches

A few other tools exist that have been used to study speech. For example, aerodynamic analysis and fiberoptic endoscopy are both routinely used in research and clinical settings in our field. However, neither has seen much direct application to the remediation of speech sound errors, and thus they are not discussed further here.

Magnetic resonance imaging (MRI) has also been used in some research applications for studying speech sound production. Similar to ultrasound, it is particularly useful for viewing soft tissues such as the tongue and velum. It also has the advantage of providing views across three dimensions. However, largely because of its cost, it is unlikely to be usable in most clinical settings at this time.

Electromagnetic articulography (EMA) is a method that makes use of magnets and evaluates movements during speech and swallowing. Data are gathered similar to the x-ray microbeam, although no ionizing radiation is involved. Small magnetic coils are attached to the articulators, and each coil emits magnetic waves of specific frequencies that are tracked by a set of magnetic sensors connected to a computer. EMA studies have provided some information on normal speech production (Goozee et al., 2007). Unfortunately, these systems remain very expensive. As such, they have seen limited application to speech remediation except in a few research settings. A few treatment studies using this technology have been conducted but have focused on adults with more significant problems (e.g., Katz et al., 1999, 2010).

TERMINOLOGY AND PHONETIC SYMBOLS

Readers are likely to have been taught using several different phonetic symbol conventions to describe /r/. For our purposes here, three specific phonetic symbols will be used. The symbol /r/[7] will be used (rather than the /ɹ/ preferred by the International Phonetic Association [IPA]) for the consonant version of this sound for three reasons: (1) our focus is on the General American English production target, (2) the symbol is consistent with English spelling, and (3) it is the phonetic symbol most commonly used for this sound by speech-language pathologists (SLPs) in the United States and Canada.

A second symbol convention to be used here follows from the assumption that this sound functions in American English as both a consonant and a vowel (but see Lockenvitz et al., 2015, for a discussion). As such, different symbols will be used. In prevocalic or initial position (whether as a singleton such as in _run_ or as a cluster as in t_ree_), this sound always serves as a consonant. The same is true in _most_ postvocalic uses. For example, it is a consonant in words such as _bear, bore, hour, beer, fire, bar,_ or _tour._ Note that in each case, it is possible to identify a separate vowel or diphthong followed by a consonant /r/. However, in words like _burr, word, hurt, third, earth, bird, church, girl, germ,_ and _surface_, it is difficult if not impossible to identify a vowel separate from the /r/ quality present. The /r/ and the vowel seem to have merged into a single sound. For our purposes, here these forms are referred to as the vocalic form, and the symbol /ɝ/ will be used when the sound occurs in stressed syllables. In unstressed syllables (as in the second syllable of _fender_ or _neighbor_), the symbol /ɚ/ will be used. To illustrate, representative words and their transcriptions are shown in Table 1–1.

---

[7]In true IPA, /r/ actually refers to a trilled form that is used elsewhere such as in Spanish, or Scottish English. That sound will _not_ be discussed here.

Table 1–1. Transcribed Examples of Words Containing Consonantal and Vocalic Forms of /r/

Prevocalic Consonant /r/		Postvocalic Consonant /r/		Stressed Vocalic /ɝ/		Unstressed Vocalic /ɚ/	
Regular Spelling	Transcription	Regular Spelling	Transcription	Regular Spelling	Transcription	Regular Spelling	Transcription
reed	/rid/	deer	/dir/	burr	/bɝ/	mayor	/mejɚ/
rent	/rɛnt/	hair	/hɛr/	turn	/tɝn/	dealer	/dilɚ/
raft	/ræft/	clear	/klir/	word	/wɝd/	dancer	/dænsɚ/
room	/rum/	spare	/spɛr/	stir	/stɝ/	super	/supɚ/
rook	/rʊk/	tour	/tur/	learn	/lɝn/	loaner	/lonɚ/
rope	/rop/	corn	/kɔrn/	flurry	/flɝi/	miter	/maɪtɚ/
rod	/rad/	car	/kar/	berg	/bɝg/	waiter	/wetɚ/
rye	/raɪ/	tire	/taɪr/	heard	/hɝd/	tower	/taʊɚ/
round	/raʊnd/	sour	/saʊr/	girl	/gɝl/	lawyer	/lɔɪjɚ/

EVIDENCE-BASED PRACTICE

As a final item to set the stage for our discussions to follow, readers may have noticed already that wherever appropriate, primary, empirical sources are being provided. This continues throughout this book because of a desire to model engaging in evidence-based practice (EBP). ASHA (2005) has mandated that we approach the work we do as SLPs from this framework. As Kamhi (2006) noted, "EBP is not simply using an intervention approach that has research support" (p. 271). It means integrating three things:

- the best available published evidence
- our clinical expertise
- patient preferences and values

It is likely that you have heard or read several discussions about what these mean; thus, I will not belabor this topic. I offer the following perspective here on how to apply it. First, note that these three elements need to be integrated. That does not mean the published evidence and clinical expertise are equal; taking that position would imply that if you have a lot of experience, you can simply ignore the published evidence. No matter how much experience you or I may have had, we have a perspective, and a point of view. That perspective is a potential form of bias. It includes a set of suppositions we have made based on our very limited view. No matter how much experience we may have had, none of us has seen it all. None of us has assessed or treated a representative sample of patients or problems. Typically, that means we have only seen those patients or problems that just happened to end up in front of us. That then means we have a set of mental blinders on that have the potential to prevent us from making the best decisions.

That said, the published evidence is also not perfect. Published evidence only tells us what *might* work. Any published treatment study provides evidence that demonstrates whether or not, with particular patients, in a particular setting, that particular approach has made a difference. It does not guarantee that it will work with the particular patient in front of you. If your patient happens to be very similar to the patients described in the study, there is a good chance that it might work for them. If your patient is very different, it does not mean it will not work. It just means you can be somewhat less certain that it will work.

It is my intention to present as much of the content here as is possible through the lens of published empirical evidence. With treatment evidence, the level of evidence needs to be considered. For our purposes, we use the evidence levels that mirror levels that have been endorsed by

ASHA, as shown in Table 1–2. These levels represent different degrees to which the research study controlled for outside influences. The higher the evidence level, the better is the control (i.e., the less likely something else might be responsible for any effect seen). Put another way, the higher the evidence, the more trust we can have in the validity of the results.

Knowing the particular level of evidence may also be quite important if there is conflicting evidence. For example, occasionally one study may indicate that a particular approach works, while another may indicate the opposite. We should put more trust in the study with the highest levels of evidence. A challenge for many clinicians is that authors of published research rarely explicitly state the level of evidence. Examining the study and comparing it to charts such as Table 1–2 may be necessary when attempting to resolve conflicting evidence.

One more word about levels of evidence: Note that "clinical experience of respected authorities" is Level IV, the lowest level of evidence. My opinion, therefore, represents the lowest form of evidence. That is why I prefer to lead with the published evidence.

Returning to the second element of EBP, clinical expertise, I have always taken this to mean our ability to demonstrate (using actual clinical data) whether the treatment currently being applied is actually making a difference with the patient we are currently treating. That means that for me, clinical expertise really means clinical evidence (also called *practice-based evidence*).

Table 1–2. Levels of Evidence

Ia	Well-designed meta-analysis of greater than one randomized control trial
Ib	Well-designed randomized control trial; includes multiple baseline designs[a]
IIa	Well-designed controlled study without randomization; includes multiple baseline designs[a]
IIb	Well-designed quasi-experimental study; includes preplanned (prospective) single subject reports that track data over time[b]
III	Well-designed nonexperimental studies (i.e., correlational and case studies)
IV	Expert committee report, consensus conference, clinical experience of respected authorities

[a]Including multiple baseline (i.e., single subject) designs is not typical, but an argument can be made that these types of studies provide as much experimental control as group designs. This is particularly the case because most group studies in speech-language pathology include relatively small numbers.

[b]Again not typical but careful data collection on individual subjects over time provides some level of control over extraneous effects, similar to planned group studies without control groups or randomization where group sizes are small.

Finally, the third element of EBP to integrate into our process is client preferences and values. As I outline in this book, there are a number of different approaches that have been shown to be effective at remediating /r/. That means there are options available to us. Under EBP, we are obliged to present the options (those that we can reasonably make use of) to the patient and/or their parents and work with them to arrive at a joint decision about how to proceed.

One option for treatment that is technically always available is no treatment. EBP requires that this be made clear. Parents generally do not refuse to allow their children to receive treatment for speech and language problems (though there are exceptions). However, much of the focus of this book is on school-age children. Although parents ultimately will be making the therapy decisions for their child, as children get older, their own preferences should also be considered. In research contexts, children above the age of 7 to 8 years are typically asked to give their "assent" or agreement to participate. If they do not agree, they cannot be compelled to participate in the study. In clinical situations, most legal experts agree that unless the treatment is necessary to save their lives or prevent serious harm, the child should have the option to refuse treatment. Most parents will acknowledge that if a child does not want to participate in therapy, the likelihood of much change happening is low. In such cases, most would tend to acquiesce to their child's wishes. In cases where the parents' preferences and the child's preferences conflict, however, guidance from local administrators should be sought.

Table 1–3 summarizes the above interpretation of EBP.

Table 1–3. Summary Interpretation of Evidence-Based Practice

Aspect to be Integrated	Interpretation
Best available published evidence	Find options regarding what MIGHT work.
Clinical expertise	Collect clinical data to see if it is ACTUALLY working.
Patient preferences and values	Present options where possible. Respect family and patient choices.

CHAPTER 2

Typical Production of American English /r/

G iven the challenges so many clinicians appear to be having with this sound, a refresher and/or update on how /r/ is produced seems appropriate. If we really want to sort out the problem, it makes sense to have a precise understanding of the goal. Although some readers will be tempted to ignore this chapter, I suspect that at least some of what is about to be presented here will be new to most.

ARTICULATORY FEATURES OF /r/

Consonant sounds are typically described relative to voicing, manner of articulation, and place of articulation. There appears to be little controversy regarding voicing and manner for American English /r/. It is generally accepted to be a voiced sound, although the possible loss of voicing in some contexts has been suggested. Its manner of articulation is listed variously as a *rhotic*, an *approximant*, or a *liquid*, and all three terms are quite appropriate. According to Ladefoged and Maddieson (1996), American English /r/ is one of several sounds belonging to the category *rhotic*. This category is unusual in phonetics in that it simply refers to those sounds that happen to be represented in spelling, when using the Latin (Roman) alphabet, by the letter "r." The terms *approximant* and *liquid* are more directly descriptive of the manner of articulation for /r/. They are somewhat synonymous terms in that both refer to a vowel-like sound in which there is only slightly more constriction in the vocal tract than for most vowels.

Three Places of Constriction (Articulation)

Adequately describing /r/ becomes complicated when defining its place of articulation. As with most speech sounds, it is the location of the narrowing or constriction for /r/ that yields its particular sound quality. As mentioned in Chapter 1, /r/ includes three different places of constriction rather than one or two seen with other sounds. It is likely that in your phonetics training, you only discussed two constrictions with the main focus for /r/ being around the constriction in the oral cavity; typically it is said to occur at the palate. However, even that description may be inadequate. If you consider the two most commonly mentioned tongue shapes for /r/ (retroflex and bunched; to be discussed later), there appear to be two somewhat different places where a narrowing of the oral cavity would be occurring: (a) near the front of the palate (just behind the alveolar ridge) for a retroflex tongue shape or (b) farther back on the palate (just in front of the velum) for a bunched tongue shape.

The second constriction that only gets passing mention in most phonetics classes is at the lips. American English /r/ is typically described as involving lip rounding (somewhat less than that seen for most English back vowels), although the amount of lip rounding for /r/ can vary greatly from one speaker to the next and from one word context to the next.

The third constriction for /r/ is often not mentioned in most undergraduate phonetics classes. This is a constriction in the pharyngeal cavity involving some degree of narrowing between the tongue root and the posterior pharyngeal wall. Although there is still not much understood about this constriction, given that at least two different tongue positions (shapes) yield the same acoustic output, at the very least speakers likely make simultaneous adjustments to both the oral and pharyngeal constrictions. This is suggested by Boyce (2015) who noted that "the pharyngeal constriction in American English speakers tends to be narrower for tongue configurations with a raised tongue tip [retroflex] and wider for tongue configurations with a 'bunched' configuration" (p. 262).

The need for and the interaction among the constrictions was also noted by Delattre and Freeman (1968):

> Experiments with an electronic analog of the mouth, which permits the shifting of constrictions and the observation of the auditory effect of each modification, have shown that the pharyngeal cavity alone does not produce an American /r/ . . . it is the palate-velar constriction which produces the American /r/ . . . as a constriction is slowly moved from the alveols [sic] toward the back, the auditory impression of the American /r/ increases, reaches a maximum near the frontier of the palate and velum and rapidly disappears beyond that point. When the palato-velar constriction is held, if the pharyngeal constriction is

narrowed, the auditory impression of /r/ is enhanced . . . if the pharyngeal constriction is widened, the /r/ is subjectively mellowed but does not disappear. (p. 42)

Ultrasound is now providing additional insight on this issue. In an ultrasound treatment study, Preston, Leece, and Maas (2017) reported that "(c)orrect productions were generally associated with elevation of the anterior tongue and depression of the tongue dorsum indicative of tongue root retraction" (p. 86). Dugan and colleagues (2019) also used ultrasound with four children to conduct a detailed analysis of movements of different parts of the tongue; they reported that the two children with normal /r/ productions used more tongue movement overall and moved individual parts of the tongue to greater degrees than the two children who produced /r/ errors. Even if ultrasound intervention remains beyond the reach of most of our patients and families, such analyses may be quite valuable. They are beginning to provide us with cuing strategies to provide to other patients (i.e., those without the benefit of ultrasound feedback) to teach them to modify those constrictions and generate acceptable /r/ productions.[1] These are discussed later.

It is in fact likely that English speakers are coordinating all three constrictions to produce a correct /r/. You may recall from your acoustics class that American English /r/ is characterized by a lowering of the value of the third formant (F3). *Perturbation theory* suggests that lowering of F3 results from a combination of all three constrictions (lips, palate, pharynx). Lindau (1985) used a combination of acoustic and x-ray data from six speakers of American English to reach a similar conclusion, noting that "it seems that speakers of American English combine all available articulatory mechanisms to produce a low third formant for /r/" (p. 163).

Gender Differences in the Constrictions for /r/

Gender differences in the acoustic characteristics of most speech sounds have been clearly documented. Those differences are typically described in terms of lower formant frequencies in males that simply reflect their overall longer vocal tracts. That said, as suggested in Chapter 1, the picture is likely more complicated. As Hagiwara (1995) reminds us, data and analysis by Fant (1963) indicated that male and female vocal tracts are actually organized (i.e., proportioned) differently. The average length of the adult male oral cavity (8.25 cm) is shorter than the average length of the corresponding male pharyngeal cavity (9.1 cm), yielding a ratio of

---

[1]Thankfully, it is not necessary to wait for those studies to be completed as ultrasound is not the only alternative approach available to remediate /r/ with evidence of effectiveness.

0.91. The average adult female oral and pharyngeal cavities are equal in length (7.0 cm each), yielding a ratio of 1.0. If the acoustic quality associated with /r/ is a function of the combination of the oral and pharyngeal constrictions, Hagiwara (1995) has suggested that males and females would need to create those constrictions in different places. In particular, he suggested that for females the oral constriction would need to be made relatively further forward in the mouth than for males.

TONGUE SHAPES FOR /r/

The idea of multiple constrictions that can be combined to generate the acoustic characteristics of /r/ implies that different combinations could be used successfully. In fact, prior to the use of ultrasound and continuing today, this has been implied by the ongoing discussion of different possible tongue shapes for an American English /r/. Phonetics textbooks (e.g., Shriberg et al., 2019) often suggest at least two such shapes: retroflex and bunched.

Might there be more than two tongue shapes for /r/? Delattre and Freeman (1968) used analysis of x-ray motion pictures from 46 adult speakers of British ($n = 3$) and American English ($n = 43$) to examine this issue. By grouping the tongue shapes they observed by visual similarity, they suggested there could be at least eight possible shapes (though only six of these were used by the speakers of American English). It is worth noting that although Delattre and Freeman included speakers from several different American dialect regions, they did not find any association between particular tongue shapes and particular dialects.

On a related note, the analysis confirmed the theoretical discussion about constrictions in both the oral and pharyngeal cavities for American English /r/. At the same time, the two shapes they associated with British English "only have ONE clear constriction, either at the pharynx . . . , or at the palate" (Delattre & Freeman, 1968, p. 42).

Another study of tongue shapes for /r/ was conducted by Westbury, Hashi, and Lindstrom (1998). In this case, they used the x-ray microbeam (see Chapter 1) to collect data from 53 American English adults, mostly from the Midwest. Tongue shapes were generated by connecting the positions of adjacent pellets using straight lines. They then calculated a set of three angles created among the four pellets and grouped them into similar shapes based on the sets of angles. Based on the pellet positions at the beginning of voicing for the /r/ in the word *row* and from the /r/ in *street*, the analysis resulted in four different tongue shapes.

Jakielski and Gildersleeve-Neumann (2018) mention that there may be three unique tongue shapes for American English /r/:

A *bunched rhotic* [emphasis added] with the tongue tip down and the highest point of the tongue raised in a mid position toward the center of the mouth or the hard palate. The back edges of the tongue touch the back molars. The *alternative tongue tip rhotic* [emphasis added] has the tongue raised midway toward the back of the hard palate and the back edge of the tongue touching the back molars. The lips are rounded. However, some speakers of English produce [ɝ] using a *retroflex tongue* [emphasis added] gesture, that is, with the tongue tip curled up and back. (pp. 83–84)

Hagiwara (1995) presented data from 15 speakers and also suggested three tongue shapes for /r/ (which he termed *tip-down, blade up, tip up*) which appear to be quite similar to the three types just highlighted from Jakielski and Gildersleeve-Neumann.

Clearly this creates a somewhat confusing picture. How many different shapes are there for American English /r/? Two? Three? Four? Six? This is clearly not a trivial question. Clinicians need to know what target shape or shapes to aim for in therapy. Although some studies of these different versions of /r/ have suggested acoustic differences among them, not all investigators report differences. It is worth noting that the studies of the shapes were all based on productions that sounded like a perfectly acceptable /r/.

Although different shapes can be identified, researchers have suggested that not all the differences are clinically relevant. Westbury and colleagues (1998) noted that "(o)bserved differences in /ɹ/ are probably not significant at levels related to categorical perception (Is this /ɹ/ or /l/?), [or] clinical assessment (Is this a 'bad' /ɹ/ requiring therapy?)" (p. 221). Likewise, a 2016 paper by Mielke, Baker, and Archangeli discussed the eight different types proposed by Delattre and Freeman (1968) and suggested that these types "are exemplars of categories and not clearly useful as prototypes" (p. 103). In other words, they may be visually different, but the differences among them may not be meaningfully different for therapy. Even if they were, with the exception of the direct visual feedback of ultrasound, which is not likely to be available to most of our patients any time soon, we are not currently able to give specific enough feedback to allow them to produce very many different tongue shapes.

Giving instructions for making the distinction between the classic categories of *retroflex* and *bunched* would seem to be much more straightforward in terms of therapy targets. The former requires that the tongue tip be raised up above the midplane of the tongue body, while the latter suggests that the tongue tip remain clearly below that midplane. In addition, the emerging evidence from the treatment options to be discussed here also implies that the distinction into two basic types should work in most cases.

> **Box 2–1**
>
> Although many tongue shapes have been proposed for /r/, assuming that there are two tongue shapes for /r/ (bunched and retroflex) remains the most practical approach.

The two classic tongue shapes (retroflex and bunched) are illustrated in Figures 2–1 and 2–2, respectively.

Which Shape Is the Most Common?

As suggested in Chapter 1, anecdotal reports suggest that clinicians tend to focus heavily on a retroflex tongue shape. There are two possible explanations for this. First, a retroflex tongue shape may be more visible in the mouth and thus may be more easily modeled and imitated. This at least potentially increases the likelihood of treatment success.[2] The second possibility is that many clinicians may simply assume that the retroflex tongue is the most commonly used shape. If it is more common, this would also increase the likelihood of success with that shape. It would also mean that it would be less likely that we would have to switch to the other shape (which may be confusing for some patients) if our first choice was not helping them to produce a correct /r/. However, starting with a retroflex /r/ target makes less sense if a bunched tongue shape is actually more common.

No large-scale studies of the frequency of /r/ tongue shapes appear to have been conducted to date, and the available reports are somewhat contradictory. Secord and colleagues (2007) commented that "the retroflex tongue shapes appear to be less common than other types across the normal population of American English speakers" (p. 142). Mielke, Baker, and Archangeli (2016) compiled findings from several studies including most of those discussed earlier. They concluded that some speakers use a retroflex shape exclusively, while others use a bunched shape exclusively. A third group uses both shapes, but some of these did so somewhat randomly, while the remainder varied their shape specifically by phonetic context (i.e., bunched more often in vocalic and postvocalic contexts and retroflex in prevocalic contexts). Mielke and colleagues then added to the available evidence using ultrasound images from 27 adult American English speakers producing /r/ in a variety of phonetic contexts. They

---

[2]It has been suggested to me that this visibility assists with establishing the sound in isolation but that some children (once /r/ is well established) spontaneously switch to a more bunched tongue shape as therapy progresses.

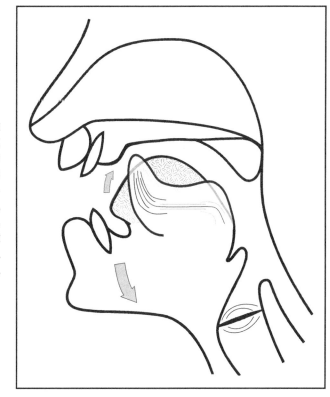

Figure 2–1. Retroflex tongue shape for /r/. From *Phonetic Science for Clinical Practice* by Kathy J. Jakielski and Christina E. Gildersleeve-Neumann, 2018, p. 85. Copyright 2018 Plural Publishing. All Rights Reserved.

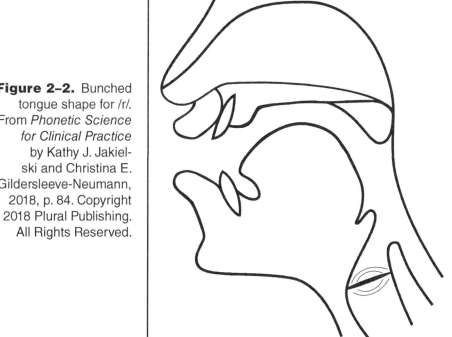

Figure 2–2. Bunched tongue shape for /r/. From *Phonetic Science for Clinical Practice* by Kathy J. Jakielski and Christina E. Gildersleeve-Neumann, 2018, p. 84. Copyright 2018 Plural Publishing. All Rights Reserved.

found that 16 of the 27 participants used only a bunched /r/, 2 used only a retroflex /r/, and the remaining 9 used both. These data would suggest that a bunched shape might be more common. Another review by Boyce, Tiede, Espy-Wilson, and Groves-Wright (2015) was conducted to examine whether dialect might influence the choice of tongue shape for /r/. They concluded that "the simplest explanation of the data reviewed here is that the choice of tongue shape for /ɹ/ is a matter of individual variation rather than regional dialect" (p. 4).

Together the available evidence does not allow us to say with any certainty that a single tongue shape is used by most speakers. Thus, it is not clear which tongue shape is going to be optimal for most patients in therapy. At the very least, clinicians need to be prepared to change the target shape if progress is limited. The need to be flexible about the choice of tongue shape to be targeted is supported by findings from an ultrasound study by McAllister Byun, Hitchcock, and Swartz (2014). These authors stated that for both ultrasound and other treatment approaches:

> It is not optimal to target a single tongue shape for all clients; instead clients should be offered opportunities to explore different tongue shapes to find the configuration that is most facilitative of perceptually accurate rhotic sounds. (p. 2128)

Box 2–2

It is not clear whether a bunched or retroflex tongue shape is more common.

Some speakers use only one version exclusively.

Other speakers vary their shape depending on the phonetic context.

TONGUE BRACING FOR /r/

Another challenge for /r/, which was mentioned in Chapter 1, is limited tactile feedback. As a liquid consonant, production of /r/ only involves a relative narrowing of the vocal tract. As such, unlike many other consonant sounds, the tongue appears to have limited contact with the rest of the vocal tract, and the amount of tactile feedback available would appear to be limited.

Limited contact does *not*, however, mean zero contact or zero tactile feedback. Some tactile feedback may actually be available. The assumption of no contact likely comes from our reliance on two-dimensional images such as those from the tracing of x-ray images; even ultrasound only gives us a two-dimensional view at any one time.[3] Thus, we seem to have been ignoring most of the rest of the tongue. It has been suggested for some time (e.g., Stone, 1990) that speakers may brace the back or sides of the tongue for much of speech. In 2013, Gick and his colleagues reviewed available electropalatography (EPG), electromagnetic articulography (EMA), and ultrasound data and concluded that this was true; speakers brace their tongues against the palate and/or jaw for almost all speech sounds. The amount of bracing likely varies by speech sound. Specific to /r/, Bacsfalvi (2010) reported that (based on coronal view ultrasound images) many speakers appear to exhibit bracing of the posterior part of the tongue against the upper molars that results in a midline groove in the tongue.

Why might this be important for /r/? Given different tongue shapes for /r/, the amount or type of bracing (and therefore the nature of any tactile feedback generated) *may* vary across those shapes. Figure 2–3 shows an EPG image and x-ray tracing for a bunched /r/. In this case, bracing is likely against the upper teeth and palate; but, bracing for a retroflex /r/ (a tongue body low within the oral cavity and minimal contact with the palate) might be against the lower teeth or jaw. An EPG image in such cases might not be very helpful as no contact would be visible.[4] The choice of which tongue shape to target in therapy would therefore mean potentially different kinds of available tactile feedback. This may account for why changing the tongue shape target may lead to success for some patients; perhaps it is at least partially because of altered tactile feedback.

One final comment relative to tongue bracing for /r/. This should not be interpreted as a total blockage of the airstream. It only anchors the tongue at the sides. Coronal (face on) views with ultrasound have shown that during production of /r/ (particularly a bunched /r/), the center of the tongue is pulled down slightly from the sides forming a central channel. Neal (2020) referred to this as a "U-shaped tongue" for /r/.

MORE THAN ONE KIND OF /r/?

Setting aside the tongue shape question, it has been suggested that one of the reasons that /r/ is both difficult to learn and difficult to remediate is that it is not just one sound. It may vary in the way it is produced

---

[3]Rotating the ultrasound probe allows for a left-to-right view of the tongue to complement the typical front-to-back view.

[4]I must confess that prior to discovering this work on tongue bracing, and prior to learning that bunched /r/ may be at least as frequent as retroflex /r/, I was convinced that EPG therapy would be pointless for /r/ because there would be limited visual feedback. As shown in Chapter 9, that was an incorrect assumption on my part.

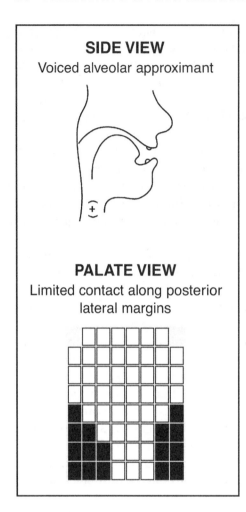

SIDE VIEW
Voiced alveolar approximant

PALATE VIEW
Limited contact along posterior
lateral margins

Figure 2–3. Tongue shape for /r/ (*upper image*) and electropalatography contact pattern (*lower image*) for a bunched /r/. From *Seeing Speech: A Quick Guide to Speech Sounds* by Sharynne McLeod and Sadanand Singh, 2009. Copyright © 2009 Plural Publishing. All Rights Reserved.

depending on the phonetic context in which it is produced. The fact that some speakers appear to use different tongue shapes in different contexts supports this. What would logically follow is that for some speakers it may be necessary to treat each phonetic context for /r/ individually.

The possibility of different versions of /r/ was implied in Chapter 1 during the discussion of the different phonetic symbols to be used for /r/. However, the different symbols being used for this sound only reflect differences in the linguistic function of /r/ within the syllable (consonant versus vowel), and its position in the word (pre- versus postvocalic for the consonant form and stressed versus unstressed syllable for the vocalic form). Acoustically, consonant and vocalic /r/ are the same (they differ primarily on duration and loudness).

Proponents of treating many different kinds of /r/ have suggested a much finer set of divisions that are based on the specific phonetic contexts in which /r/ might occur. One example of such a set of divisions (adapted from Ristuccia, 2002) is shown in Table 2–1.

The argument for different types of /r/ appears to be based on the idea that the surrounding contexts can influence how it is produced. There is little dispute about this. Context matters for /r/ as it does for every other speech sound. For example, consider /s/. When produced before a rounded vowel, speakers often round their lips during the production even though lip rounding is not usually associated with /s/. However, when /s/ is produced before an unrounded vowel, there is typically no lip rounding. Likewise, in faster, more casual speech, front or back vowels tend to be produced closer to the center of the vowel space than if they were being produced by themselves or in slower, careful speech (also called *clear* speech). All of these adjustments are examples of what is called *coarticulation,* which represents our very natural tendency to make the process of speaking more efficient. The ideal movement patterns for sounds spoken in isolation are modified to take into account where the articulators have come from and/or where they will be going next. Put another way, we take shortcuts when we produce a sound in the context of other sounds. We do so because this allows us to produce speech more quickly and with less

Table 2–1. Different Types of /r/

Context	Example Word	Context	Example Word
/ɝ/ initial	earth	/or/ medial	cork
/ɝ/ medial	fern	/or/ final	door
/ɝ/ final	fur	/ir/ initial	ear
Prevocalic (initial) /r/	red	/ir/ medial	zero
/ɚ/ medial	perform	/ir/ final	deer
/rl/ medial	Charlie	/ɛr/ initial	airplane
/rl/ final	girl	/ɛr/ medial	fairy
/ɑr/ initial	art	/ɛr/ final	hair
/ɑr/ medial	barn	/ɑɪr/ initial	Ireland
/ɑr/ final	far	/ɑɪr/ medial	fireplace
/or/ initial	organ	/ɑɪr/ final	tire

Note. Adapted from *The Entire World of R Instructional Workbook: A Phonemic Approach to /r/ Remediation* by C. Ristuccia, 2002. Say It Right. Copyright 2002 by Say It Right.

effort. We also likely do so because we can get away with it; there is little effect on our listeners (i.e., they usually do not notice), and communication is rarely affected. However, the idea that every phonetic context creates a unique sound form that must be learned (and by extension taught in therapy) only seems to have been applied to /r/.

Is /r/ a special case? Does its complexity (e.g., those three different constrictions to be coordinated) mean that the amount of motor learning required is simply greater than for other sounds? Do some speakers need to focus on each very specific context one at a time in order to master /r/? Maybe. The implication is that the mixing of contexts that we typically do in therapy may be too confusing for some children. Perhaps some of them need to work with a much narrower set of contexts to allow them to learn the sound. Two general observations support this notion. First, some children come to us with what at first appears to be inconsistent accuracy. In some of these cases, however, if we take the time to examine the specific contexts of /r/, we discover that they are consistently correct in some contexts and consistently incorrect in some other contexts. Such children might benefit from treating /r/ as more than one sound. Second, recall the previous discussion on the frequency of different tongue shapes for /r/. The fact that some speakers vary the tongue shape they use for /r/ depending on the phonetic context suggests that they are treating it as several sounds.

These observations, however, do not prove that such an approach would be effective in therapy. What is needed is direct empirical evidence showing that a narrow focus on specific contexts helps some children learn /r/. Clinicians using this approach report anecdotally that it appears to work, but there does not appear to have been any published studies of the use of the different kinds of /r/ listed in Table 2–1. Two older studies do provide some related findings. Both looked at whether a narrow focus on one particular form of /r/ might lead to generalization to other forms. In both cases, the three versions of /r/ discussed in Chapter 1 (/r/, /ɝ/, /ɚ/) were used. Elbert and McReynolds (1975) treated 12 children aged 6 to 11 years using traditional sound shaping therapy three times per week for 10 to 15 min. Findings indicated that "(m)ost subjects increased the number of correct responses to untrained items in several allophonic categories regardless of the specific allophone taught" (p. 386). Hoffman (1983) conducted a similar study with 12 children age 5;6 to 7;10 who received sound shaping therapy twice a week for 30 min. The outcomes were similar. All children generalized to untrained forms of /r/ regardless of which form was trained. Together these findings suggest that a narrow focus on either consonantal or vocalic /r/ may help *some* children master this sound. Perhaps limiting our treatment focus to one particular context may help some children.

As appealing as the prospect is of jumping in and working on each narrow phonetic context one at a time might be, a caveat is in order.

Although it may work for some patients, using such an approach may prove counterproductive. It may actually limit motor learning. In Chapter 5, principles of motor learning are discussed. One of these involves the idea that we should practice speech sound targets in a variety of contexts to encourage automaticity or flexibility. The ultimate goal for all of our patients is that they should be able to produce any speech sound in any valid phonetic context whenever they need to do so. Sticking too narrowly or for too long to specific contexts may actually discourage such flexibility; it risks therapy becoming the learning of particular motor patterns by rote (the exact opposite of flexibility). Mixing a variety of different contexts into our therapy needs to happen at some point to encourage flexibility in motor planning and motor execution.

CHAPTER 3

When to Intervene

There are at least two broad perspectives that clinicians use to decide when intervention should occur for /r/ or for any other sound. Some use one perspective exclusively over the other, while many use some combination of the two.

DEVELOPMENTAL LOGIC

For most clinicians, the answer to the question about when to intervene is fairly straightforward: We should do so when the child is producing errors past the age when most children would have already mastered it. This is what I refer to as *developmental logic*. It assumes that all children learning the same language are working with the same basic neural architecture and the same basic articulatory structures, and that their brains all process information in essentially the same way. As such, speech sound acquisition should proceed in the same order for all children. With children who are behind where we expect them to be, the goal is to help them to catch up by starting with the thing on which they are the furthest behind and then targeting the thing that was next furthest behind, and so on. The goal is effectively to try to bring them back into line with the sequence of typical development. To put it another way, developmental logic means the order of things for therapy should be the same as the order in typical development. Using the same logic, therapy is justified only when a child is either clearly behind or not following the normal developmental sequence.

THE NORMATIVE DATA

Following developmental logic for treating any sound then requires knowing when that sound is typically mastered (i.e., at what age are most children using it correctly?). There remains some debate about when exactly that occurs for /r/.

Defining Mastery

Although there are many sources of information that can help us answer the mastery question, unfortunately they do not agree on the age at which /r/ is mastered (this is true for almost all speech sounds). The disagreements arise mostly from the fact that the sources did not all try to answer the mastery question the same way. There is some agreement in at least one respect, namely, that all reported data from the production of single words. Although single word production may not be fully representative of what speakers do in their everyday speech, at least there is a common basis for comparison. However, that is where the similarities seem to end. Almost all of the sources selected their own unique sets of words. The net result is variations in the surrounding phonetic contexts in which /r/ was embedded. The sources also differed relative to where in the word /r/ was positioned. Using the classic initial, medial, and final word positions, some included all three positions, while others included only initial and final positions. Several sources only reported findings for initial position. Some sources tested /r/ at more than one word position but reported findings collapsed across positions. Finally, even though each source used relatively large samples, each tested a different group of children.

In terms of the criterion they used for mastery, the sources were also not in full agreement. Most reported findings on the age at which 90% of children are correctly producing /r/. Some used lower cutoffs (85%, 75%), and some reported more than one cutoff. The lowest cutoff reported was 50% of children.

The sources date back to at least the 1930s. These include peer-reviewed studies published in journals as well as the normative studies used to develop single word articulation tests. All were cross-sectional in nature, which means that they sampled a large group of children of varying ages all at the same time (each participant was tested only once). Various attempts have been made over the years to reconcile the data in these sources (e.g., Sander, 1972; Smit, 1986). The most comprehensive such attempt appears to be that of Crowe and McLeod (2020) who included a specific analysis of American English /r/. That analysis did not present its own data but rather compiled the data across 15 different sources and generated average ages of acquisition. This analysis then represented almost 19,000 American children.

Singleton /r/

The majority of data are available for /r/ as a singleton (i.e., by itself without any other consonants next to it in the same syllable). Rather than attempt to review each of the studies, the summary of the review by Crowe and McLeod (2020) is reproduced in Figure 3–1.

In Figure 3–1, findings for each source are represented by lines and/or dots. The left end of the line indicates the age at which 50% of children have mastered /r/. The right end of the line indicates the age at which 90% of children have mastered /r/. The dot indicates the age at which 75% of children have mastered /r/. As shown, the age of mastery for /r/ was quite variable across the sources. Using the 90% criterion, for example, values ranged from 2;6 to 8;0 (30–96 months). Crowe and McLeod (2020) computed average values across all the sources and reported three different ages for /r/ acquisition depending on the mastery criterion:

50% of children	35.40 months (2;11)
75% of children	47.64 months (4;0)
90% of children	66.58 months (5;7)

It should be noted that Crowe and McLeod (2020) did not examine gender differences in acquisition of consonants in general or /r/ in particular. An informal review of the data in the sources for /r/ suggests no gender differences for the age of mastery for /r/ in singletons.

Mastery of /r/ in Consonant Clusters

Although it is commonly assumed that consonants produced as singletons are mastered before those same consonants produced next to other consonants in the same syllable (i.e., in consonant clusters), it is worth asking whether this is specifically true for /r/. An early study by Curtis and Hardy (1959) presented some data that appeared to challenge conventional wisdom for /r/ clusters. That study tested 30 children aged 5;6 to 8;6 who had speech errors on multiple sounds including /r/. They reported that "in every instance the [r]s occurring in consonant blends were correctly articulated relatively more often than the single [r]s" (p. 250).

At least six of the sources from Figure 3–1 as well as one study that focused only on clusters provide data on age of mastery for /r/ clusters.

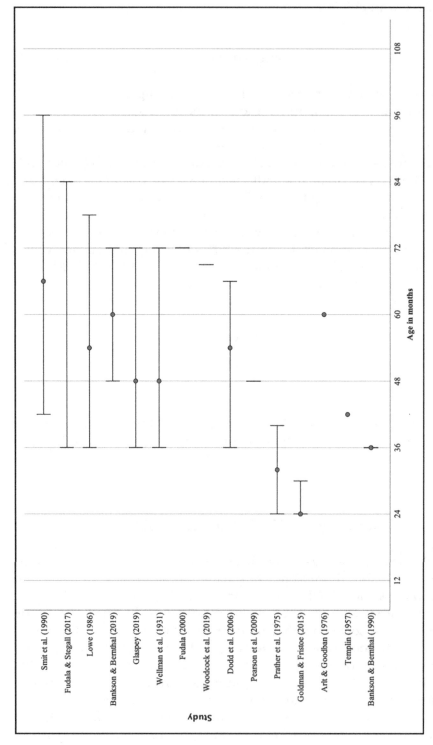

Figure 3–1. Mean age of acquisition for American English /r/ across studies from the United States (total *N* = 18,907) at 50% criterion (*low bar*), 75% criterion (*circle*), and 90% criterion (*high bar*). Studies are ordered according to mean age of acquisition at the 90% criterion. Copyright © 2020 Crowe and McLeod. All Rights Reserved. Reprinted with permission.

Note that the focus was primarily on initial position, and these are highlighted in Table 3–1. With one exception (Dawson & Tattersall, 2001), the sources reported findings using a 90% of children criterion.

As with singleton /r/, Table 3–1 yields quite variable findings. Overall the ages for mastery ranged from 4;6 to 9;0. Using the same approach as Crowe and McLeod (2020), when averaged across sources and clusters, the average age of mastery was 79 months (6;7). This represents about 1 year older than the 90% value obtained by Crowe and McLeod for age of mastery for /r/ singletons (5;7). As such, it would appear that /r/ follows the conventionally held pattern (i.e., clusters mastered later than singletons).

Most of the studies reported different ages of mastery depending on which other consonant(s) was combined with /r/. As can be seen in Table 3–1, there is no clear pattern regarding which specific /r/ clusters are mastered earlier or later than others. Note that only two sources reported separate findings by gender and only the data from Goldman and Fristoe (2015) indicate gender differences. Overall, this would suggest that similar to singleton /r/, there are likely no gender differences for mastery of /r/ clusters.

Box 3–1

Available data suggest the following mastery criteria:

/r/ singletons are mastered by 90% of children by about age 6 years

/r/ clusters are mastered by 90% of children by about age 7 years

there do not appear to be any gender differences in mastery of /r/

ALTERNATIVES TO DEVELOPMENTAL LOGIC

Following developmental logic is a reasonable approach in most instances. However, there are some valid justifications for not doing so. The first reason would be if a young child is experiencing significant negative social consequences (e.g., bullying, severe teasing) for producing errors in their speech. As discussed in Chapter 1, many clinicians would see this as a good reason to intervene in general. It might also be a valid reason to intervene earlier than we might have otherwise.

Table 3–1. Findings for Age of Mastery of /r/ in Initial Consonant Clusters[a]

Cluster	Bowers and Huisingh (2010)	Dawson and Tattersall (2001)[b]	Fudala and Stegall (2017)	Glaspey (2019)[c]	Goldman and Fristoe (2015)		McLeod and Arciuli (2009)	Smit et al. (1990)	
					Females	Males		Females	Males
/pr/	6;0–6;5				5;0–5;11	7;0–7;11	8;0	8;0	8;0
/br/	6;0–6;5	5;6			4;6–4;11	6;0–6;11	8;0	8;0	8;0
/tr/	7;0–7;5	5;6	6;0–6;5	6;0	4;6–4;11	6;0–6;11	8;0	8;0	8;0
/dr/	7;0–7;5	5;6			5;0–5;11	6;0–6;11	8;0	8;0	8;0
/kr/	7;0–7;5	5;6			5;0–5;11	6;0–6;11	8;0	8;0	8;0
/gr/	7;0–7;5		6;0–6;5		5;0–5;11	6;0–6;11	8;0	8;0	8;0
/fr/	7;0–7;5				4;6–4;11	7;0–7;11	8;0	8;0	8;0
/r/							9;0	9;0	9;0
/spr/							7;0–9;0	7;0–9;0	7;0–9;0
/str/							7;0–9;0	7;0–9;0	7;0–9;0
/skr/							7;0–9;0	7;0–9;0	7;0–9;0

[a]Cell entries are years;months, and all are based on criterion of 90% of children producing it correctly (except as indicated).
[b]Based on criterion of 85% of children producing it correctly.
[c]Based on criterion of 90% of children producing it spontaneously correctly in words (item score of 10 or better).

A second justification for not following developmental logic (and intervening earlier) is based on a desire to avoid the development of strongly ingrained bad habits (one of the challenges identified in Chapter 1). The longer and more often a motor pattern is practiced, the harder it becomes to change. As discussed in Box 3–2, some children start producing a distorted /r/ as preschoolers, but their speech overall is quite intelligible, and they often do not qualify for therapy using developmental logic. They might come to our attention later and would be labeled as having "persistent" errors. For these children, by the time they typically become eligible for therapy, they have had several years of practicing those distortion errors. Children with multiple errors as preschoolers tend to have more substitution errors ([w] for /r/), and if they fail to fully master /r/, they often transition to a distortion error. In this case, they may have had less time practicing those errors. These latter children are said to have "residual" errors.

The notion of intervening early for preschoolers who present with /r/ distortion errors (rather than substitutions) is supported by findings in

---

Box 3–2: Persistent Versus Residual Errors

The distortion errors that are seen in older children on school-based caseloads appear to come from two different histories (Flipsen, 2015):

Persistent errors: distortion errors that appear in the preschool years, but early speech was overall quite intelligible. Therapy would not have been indicated at that time. As a consequence, those early errors become ingrained. These are usually only identified as needing intervention after about age 7 to 8 years.

Residual errors: distortion errors that appear somewhat later (often as replacements for earlier substitution errors). Early speech included many errors and was quite unintelligible. Therapy began early, but these errors remain as leftovers.

It is not clear which occur more often or whether these errors respond differently to therapy, but at least one study has suggested that at age 8 years, even though both persistent and residual errors are identified as similar sounding distortions, the persistent errors are acoustically further from normal than residual errors (Shriberg et al., 2001).

Smit (1993), who reported the frequency of error types in the data from the Iowa–Nebraska norms study (Smit et al., 1990). Table 4 in the Smit (1993) paper (p. 539) shows that [w] for /r/ substitutions in initial and medial positions are common in children under age 4 years, but derhotacized productions (distortions partway between /w/ and /r/) occurred less than 15% of the time. Thus, it might make sense to intervene for the preschool child who is producing /r/ distortions.

A final justification for ignoring developmental logic relates to a somewhat uncommon but not unheard of situation. In this case, a young child with several errors qualifies for services by virtue of a score on a standardized test (i.e., a single word articulation test), but none of the speech errors qualifies as a therapy target using developmental logic. The choice in such cases is either to take a *watch and see* approach with no immediate therapy or ignore the developmental sequence and choose error targets using some other criterion (e.g., most stimulable, most frequent in the language, unusual error patterns). The fact that they are producing enough errors overall to qualify for services supports the idea of ignoring developmental logic to choose therapy targets.

Regardless of the justification for ignoring developmental logic and intervening earlier, most clinicians would take a fairly conventional approach and target /r/ using the three basic forms outlined in Chapter 1 (/r, ɝ, ɚ/). This would be followed later by targeting different /r/ clusters. An alternative might be to take the individual forms shown in Table 2–1 one at a time using an approach such as is discussed in Ristuccia (2002). At least one other alternative is available, which has received some attention. It is perhaps the ultimate counterperspective to following developmental logic. It is known as the complexity approach and was developed based on the intermingling of several linguistic theories. It is generally discussed relative to children with multiple speech sound errors, but, in principle, one might apply it to /r/. This approach presumes that, rather than working from the simplest (earliest developing) targets to more complex (later developing) targets, the opposite approach may work better. It presumes that using the most complex treatment targets will provide for greater generalization across a child's speech sound system. Explaining the underlying basis for this approach is beyond the scope of the current book, but the interested reader is referred to Storkel (2018) for an excellent discussion and several hypothetical examples. There is some research evidence supporting such an approach (e.g., Gierut, 1990, 1991), although there is also some counterevidence (Rvachew & Nowak, 2001). The possibility of using this for a child with /r/ errors is illustrated by the case example (referred to as Child 1) from Storkel (2018). The child had errors on /θ, ð, r/ and was not stimulable for any of them. The analysis concluded by suggesting that appropriate targets might include /br/, /dr/, or /gr/. However, reaching that conclusion using the complexity perspective requires a somewhat complicated analysis. The same conclusion could have been reached with much less effort by referring to the fact that, from a motor perspective, these three clusters are known to be facilitating contexts for /r/ (this is discussed in Chapter 6). Thus, it would be difficult to justify taking the complexity approach for a child with only one or two errors. However, such an approach to target selection might be quite appropriate for a child with many more speech errors.

CHAPTER 4

Assessment of /r/

This chapter focuses on several assessment issues. It includes a discussion and suggestions for identifying the nature of the problem. Few would argue that this is what should drive our treatment choices. There is also a discussion of factors to be considered in the diagnosis. Finally, some specific assessment procedures are presented.

SUBSTITUTION VERSUS DISTORTION ERRORS AND /r/

Although discussed to some extent in previous chapters, it is important to be clear about the types of errors being discussed here. As data provided by Smit (1993) indicate, the classic [w] for /r/ substitution error (e.g., saying "wabbit" for "rabbit") is common in children under age 4 years. For children who do not fully master /r/ by the time they reach second or third grade, a small percentage may continue the [w] substitution, but in most cases their error changes. It shifts to a distortion that is neither /w/ nor /r/. It is effectively partway between the two; this distortion is sometimes called a *derhotacized* /r/; this term emphasizes that the sound has lost much of its /r/-like quality. (It is not much of a rhotic anymore.) For most children, this shift from substitution to distortion happens gradually over several years. For the children in this group, who had multiple sounds in error early on and received therapy as preschoolers, the errors that remain in second or third grade are those with the residual errors discussed in Chapter 3. Smit (1993) also provided data showing that for a small subset of children under age 4 years (up to 15%), the distortion shows up at that early age. Because many of these children have few if any other errors as preschoolers, little or no concern is raised about the distortion error at that time. As they reach third or fourth grade, these errors may suddenly come to our attention, but they have been there all along and represent highly overpracticed forms. These children represent those with the "persistent" errors discussed in Chapter 3.

A related consideration for /r/ errors involves what happens in word final position. In this position, distorted /r/ will still be distorted, but the speaker who substitutes [w] in another word position will not do so in final position. This is because as a glide consonant, the phoneme /w/ never occurs in a word final position (it represents a transition between two other sounds). Although many words may be spelled with the letter "w," if you examine all such words (e.g., fellow, hollow, pillow, view, flow, raw, new, vow, bow, cow), you will notice that they actually all end in back vowels or diphthongs. Because /w/ cannot be used, speakers who would normally substitute [w] for /r/ in other word positions will end up substituting a back vowel or diphthong. A word like car becomes /kɑo/, deer becomes /dio/, and air becomes /ɛo/.

Knowing whether a distorted /r/ is a residual or a persistent error can be important in therapy because it helps us understand how long the distortion has been practiced and how much of a habit needs to be overcome. However, for assessment purposes, there is no practical difference between a persistent /r/ error and a residual /r/ error. As distortions, they sound the same. A detailed acoustic analysis may be able to separate the two (see Shriberg et al., 2001), but such an analysis is not practical in most clinical situations. The vast majority of clinicians will rely on their ears, and even very experienced clinicians cannot hear the difference between them. They are both simply distortions. Only an examination of the child's case history would allow us to differentiate the two types.

Transcribing and Scoring Productions

In Chapter 1, included in the challenges discussed regarding /r/ were the "constraints of categorical perception." Most listeners, including some clinicians, do not immediately notice distortion errors because of our very natural tendency to want to fit what we hear into a specific phoneme category. With /r/ errors, they tend to get labeled as either /w/ or /r/. Although for most listeners the distinction is not all that important, separating distortions from substitutions clearly is important for clinical practice. As discussed later in this chapter, the distinction will both help define the nature of the problem and offer some direction for remediation.

Separating a [w] of /r/ substitution from a distorted /r/ consistently requires some practice. A study by Klein and colleagues (2012), for example, showed that inexperienced clinicians were quite good at identifying correct /r/ productions but were quite variable in their ability to separate out error types. Thus, for readers with either limited experience or for those who are concerned about their ability to hear the difference, I would strongly encourage you to gain as much practice as possible with listening to and judging various productions. The SAILS app (Rvachew & Herbay, 2017), discussed later in this chapter, can provide you with the opportunity to do that. You might also go to Dr. Jonathan Preston's website (http://www.haskins.yale.edu/PT/), where there are opportunities to practice listening to normal and error productions of several speech sounds including /r/.

THE NATURE OF THE PROBLEM

Effective therapy requires three things:

- Understanding the precise nature of the problem. That is the focus here.

- Choosing the appropriate therapy. The available options are more varied than they used to be. Several later chapters discuss the various available options.

- Proper application of the appropriate therapy. Regardless of the therapy chosen, our understanding of how to organize therapy efficiently has improved considerably. This is addressed in Chapter 6.

   Most clinicians assume that the child with a single speech sound error has an articulation problem. Given that these are typically distortion errors, this is not an unreasonable assumption. These children appear to understand what sound they are aiming for but are having difficulty with precision of movement (i.e., consistently getting the articulators into the correct configuration). However, if that were the only problem, why do some of these children fail to respond to traditional therapy? One reason might be a related issue that has been largely ignored. What about speech perception?

The /r/ Error as a Perceptual Problem

Prior to the 1960s, it was widely assumed that difficulty with speech perception was an underlying problem for most speech sound disorders. As outlined by Van Riper (1954), ear training or discrimination training was considered an integral part of speech sound therapy. However, when a number of researchers began to investigate the relationship between perception and production, a consensus eventually emerged that children with speech sound disorders do not consistently differ from their typically speaking peers on general tests of speech perception. This led many clinicians to abandon speech perception testing. Given the growing demands on clinical time, this made sense. Why engage in needless testing?

This may, however, have been a case where the baby was thrown out with the bathwater, particularly for older children with persistent and residual errors. The interested reader is referred to a review by Cabbage (2015) for a general discussion. Although children with speech sound disorders, as a group, do not appear to have perceptual problems, it has been demonstrated that speech perception difficulties may be present *for some speech production errors for some children*. For example, a child may have production errors on five or six sounds but may have a perceptual problem for only one of those sounds. In other words, for that one sound (but not any of the others), they either do not notice or have trouble hearing the difference between the target sound and the error they produce in its place. Findings from a study by Shuster (1998) suggest that this may be true for some children who produce /r/ errors. That study included 26 children age 7;1 to 13;11 (four children produced errors on at least one other sound). Half of the group had just started therapy, and the other half had been in therapy (without success) for at least 2 years. When listening to a tape recording of their own productions (some of which had been acoustically corrected), these children could not consistently identify whether their own errors were correct or not (performing at about chance levels).

Findings from two treatment studies offer some additional evidence. Wolfe, Presley, and Mesaris (2003) compared traditional articulation training with and without perception training in a group of nine preschool children with a variety of speech sound errors. Findings showed that the addition of perception training led to faster improvement but only for those errors where the child also had difficulty with perception before therapy started. Little difference was observed for errors where there was no pretreatment difficulty with perception. As well, in a study using ultrasound with and without the addition of perception training specific to /r/, Preston, Hitchcock, and Leece (2020) treated 38 children aged 8 to 16 years. They reported that "perceptual acuity was significantly related to change in /ɪ/ production accuracy" (p. 451). Greater ability to perceive their errors before treatment tended to translate to greater success in production therapy.

Taken together, this evidence suggests that perceptual deficits might account for at least some of the limited success in therapy for some children. Testing each error to determine if there is a specific perception problem with that particular sound might be worthwhile. Doing so for the child with only one or two errors such as /r/ should not pose a major burden on our time.

To be clear, this is not an either/or situation. With a perceptual problem, the child would not have a solid internal mental image of the sound and thus would not have been able to figure out the correct way to produce the sound. Although improving speech perception for particular errors is unlikely to be sufficient on its own, helping the child to finally sort out what the target is supposed to sound like may be the crucial missing piece (along with production training) for mastery of production for some children.

Box 4–1

Speech perception is the ability to distinguish the difference between speech sounds.

This is *not* the same as a hearing loss.

Most children with speech sound disorder, including those with perceptual problems, usually pass a standard hearing screening.

They may, however, have trouble hearing the difference *between some sounds*.

The /r/ Error as a Phonological Problem

It is hard to argue that distortion errors, by themselves, are anything but an articulation problem. However, in those cases where the child continues to substitute [w] for /r/ (rather than producing a distortion), another possibility needs to be considered. Here the underlying problem may be either phonological or articulatory or both. A phonological problem is a language problem. Individuals with a phonological problem have not fully sorted out the sound system (phonology) of the language. What is stored in their brains relative to the sounds of the language does not fully match what is stored in the brains of competent adult users of the language. They have what linguists call a poorly developed underlying representation.

Being able to correctly produce speech sounds in a consistent way requires a strong connection among three things: what the phoneme sounds like (the perceptual piece discussed earlier), what it feels like when it is physically produced (the articulatory or motor piece to be discussed in Chapter 5), and how that sound functions in the language (i.e., the phonological piece; how that sound is used to generate meaning). If the child produces a completely different phoneme than the target, there is a possibility that they do not fully understand what sound is supposed to be used. They may well have an incorrect underlying representation.

There is actually no straightforward way to sort out whether a speech sound error reflects a phonological or an articulatory problem. Many clinicians assume that a phonological pattern (also called "process") analysis is sufficient. Unfortunately, calling a [w] for /r/ substitution "gliding" or "liquid gliding" only just describes the error. It does not, by itself, tell us what is stored in the language system and it does not confirm that some sort of mental operation has occurred that alters what the child will produce.

At the moment, our best evidence for phonological problems is mostly indirect. It shows up in the problems some of these children have with reading and writing. The connection is not hard to make. During reading and writing with an alphabetic language like English, it is necessary to translate back and forth between the spoken and written forms. This presumes an intact underlying representation for the sound (the spoken form). If you do not fully appreciate what the spoken sound is, how can you match it to the written symbol that is supposed to represent it? A review by Farquharson (2019) identified a number of problems children with speech sound disorders may have with reading-related skills such as poor phonological awareness (e.g., Gernand & Moran, 2007), poor phonological working memory (e.g., Farquharson et al., 2017), and poor phonological processing skills such as difficulty with nonword repetition (e.g., Preston & Edwards, 2007). If none of these problems are apparent, it is likely that the problem is only articulatory.

As with perceptual problems, this is not necessarily an either/or situation. The child's difficulty with the underlying representation for the sound may be creating some confusion and interfering with their mastery of the physical production of the sound. Thus, a motor-only focus may fall short in correcting the production error, because they are attempting to match the production with an incorrect underlying form. Fortunately, phonological therapy for speech sounds requires production practice, so it effectively works on both articulatory and phonological problems at the same time.

More Than One Problem?

The earlier discussion was meant to suggest that distorted /r/ production errors are clearly articulatory, and teaching correct production is usually needed. Children with these errors as well as those who substitute [w] for /r/ may have a perceptual problem at the same time. The child who also has difficulty with reading and writing (whether they substitute or distort /r/) may also have a phonological problem.

FACTORS TO CONSIDER

Before discussing the specifics of the diagnosis, there are a number of relevant factors that should be considered.

Dialect

Some dialects of English such as many British English dialects, a stereo-typical New York or Bostonian dialect, and a classic southern U.S. dialect have been described as r-deleting (McAllister Byun & Campbell, 2016). In such dialects, vocalic and postvocalic /r/ lose much of their /r/ color, and attempts at those contexts may be perceived as derhotacized. As a part of the normal dialect being used by their speech community, such differences would not normally warrant remediation. In deciding whether such productions might need to be corrected, performance on /r/ in initial position should be examined. Speakers of most American English r-deleting dialects would typically produce a fully realized (i.e., not derhotacized) /r/ in word initial position. For speakers of those dialects, remediation would typically only be appropriate if errors were observed in initial position.

Case History

Something that is often glossed over with older children with single sound errors is their case history. There are, however, at least two reasons why the case history may be especially relevant. First, for children with distortion errors, there is the question of whether the child has previously been in therapy and for how long. As discussed previously and in Chapter 3, the child who has a long therapy history is more likely to have a residual error and may not have been practicing their distortion as long as the child with a persistent error who has had little to no time in therapy. The child with persistent errors may therefore need either more intensive therapy (if that is possible) or may need to be in therapy for an overall longer period to correct their error. Likewise, a more highly structured approach to generalization may be necessary.

The second reason for paying attention to case history for these children is the question of middle ear history. At least 30% of children experience multiple middle ear infections as preschoolers. In most cases, they grow out of it by the time they hit school age. However, during these episodes, these children may have experienced frequent periods of moderate hearing loss, and it was occurring during the critical period of speech sound acquisition. When we see them at age 7 years and older, they may be able to hear the difference between certain speech sounds, but because of their history of intermittent hearing loss, what is stored is their long-term memory for some speech sounds may be incorrect. Ear infections that occur when children are 12 to 18 months old may be especially detrimental (Shriberg et al., 2000). That means that children with histories of lots of middle ear infections and/or those who experience them in the second year of life may be especially susceptible to perceptual problems.

The Role of Stimulability

Most clinicians examine stimulability (i.e., they test whether the child can correctly imitate a production following a model) as part of their assessment process. They then assume that the child who is easily stimulable for their error, especially if they are stimulable to at least the word level, must have a phonological rather than an articulatory problem. Some children with distortion errors on /r/ are quite stimulable. The same is true for some children who substitute [w] for /r/. These children clearly can produce the sound and it may not be necessary to teach them how to produce it. The research is generally supportive of this position. Some clinicians also go so far as to suggest that the child who is stimulable for their error is very likely to master the sound on their own. While this may be true for many preschool children, it is probably not a safe assumption for school-age children with speech errors. They have been practicing their error for an extended period and have habits that can be difficult to overcome.

The older child who is stimulable may not need much specific instruction on how to physically produce the sound. However, they almost certainly will need assistance with consistently producing the correct sound, as well as generalization beyond the word level and to other situations. This is discussed in Chapter 5 as well as in the chapters related to specific treatment approaches.

Hearing Acuity

Although most children with speech sound disorders, regardless of the number of errors, pass a standard hearing screening, not all of them will. The typical practice of screening hearing should be continued for children with /r/ errors. If a hearing screening has not been conducted recently, it should be carried out. If they fail the screening, they should be referred for a full audiological evaluation.

Language Comprehension

Being able to hear the instructions or the stimuli is one thing, but does the client understand the meaning of what we are attempting to communicate to them? Can they follow our directions? Can they meaningfully relate to the stimuli being presented? These questions highlight the fact that it is also important to have a sense of the client's language comprehension skills. Reduced comprehension skills would mean, at the very least, a need to adjust any instructions that are provided. It might also limit some of the therapy options as clients with reduced comprehension skill may not be able to fully benefit from some of the more instrumental approaches such as visual acoustic feedback or electropalatography (discussed in later chapters).

Structural Issues

A standard oral–facial examination should be carried out even for a child with just /r/ errors. There may be structural issues that are interfering with their ability to produce the sound. Some of these may need to be addressed through medical referral.

Tongue-tie or ankyloglossia is one such issue. As recently as the 1970s, it was common practice for this to be surgically corrected immediately after birth. However, that is no longer the case, as it has been shown that many individuals have this condition but have normal speech. They appear to be able to compensate for the abnormal structure. The surgery, although minor, is seen as largely unnecessary (except in cases where feeding is impacted). The more typical practice now is that it is noted on the chart by the obstetrician with a comment such as "let's wait to see how speech develops." Children with /r/ errors combined with tongue-tie may be a subgroup for whom the tongue-tie is making a difference. They may be unable to adequately elevate the tip of the tongue to produce a retroflex tongue shape, thus limiting their options. Although a bunched tongue shape remains an option in most cases, it is also possible that the overall restriction in tongue movement caused by the tongue-tie may make it difficult to create the pharyngeal constriction. Parents of these children should at least be advised to consult with their pediatrician.

Chronically enlarged tonsils is another issue that may be relevant to /r/ errors. A real case will illustrate. I recall seeing a 9-year-old boy who had strong academic skills but produced /r/ distortions. The oral–facial examination revealed tonsils about the size of small plums. He was able to produce a good /r/ with a model, but when he did so he complained of a strong urge to vomit. It seemed that the retraction of the tongue root was pushing the tonsils back against the faucial pillars and eliciting a gag reflex. His parents were advised to consult an otolaryngologist to discuss the possibility of having the tonsils removed. In the end the family decided against it, and therapy was discontinued. His speech was fully intelligible, he was not affected academically, and neither he nor his parents were bothered by the error. The family was also advised that since tonsils typically peak in size around puberty and then recede, therapy for this boy might be less challenging for him when he was a teenager.

Palate structure (width and height) may or may not be relevant for /r/. Recall the previous discussion about minimal contact between the tongue and the palate (or the back teeth) during production of /r/. This suggests that all but the most extremely narrow or extremely shallow palates would have little impact on the learning or production of /r/. From a practical perspective, even if structural differences in the palate were affecting the ability to learn to produce /r/, the serious nature of any surgical correction would likely not be considered in most cases.

Relative to the teeth, with the exception of the molar teeth, they play a limited role in the production of /r/. Thus, most anomalies of the teeth are likely to have minimal impact on the learning of /r/.

Tongue Growth Patterns

In a 1982 continuing education presentation on the oral–facial examination, Robert Mason noted that the tongue grows most rapidly between age 4½ and 6 years. Assuming this to be true, working on /r/ during this period may actually prove to be counterproductive. With limited tactile feedback during production of /r/, the majority of the feedback comes from our sense of the tongue's position in space (proprioception) and movement (kinesthesis). If tongue size is changing rapidly due to rapid growth, it may be difficult for the child to keep track of what tongue position results in a good /r/ as the feedback may change from day to day. Fortunately, most clinicians follow developmental logic, and as discussed in Chapter 3, intervention for /r/ errors would not usually be indicated much before age 6 years. However, as discussed in Chapter 3, it is certainly possible to justify working on /r/ before this age. Doing so potentially moves therapy into that period of rapid tongue growth described by Mason. When this is done, and if Mason is correct, a failure to make progress with *some* children would not be surprising.

Motor Issues

Assessment of speech motor skills is a standard part of most assessments. However, excluding those with childhood apraxia or other documented motor speech disorders, there is only limited evidence available that children with speech sound disorders have poorer speech motor skills than their typically speaking peers. At least two types of evidence are relevant here. First, studies using diadochokinetic (DDK) rate tasks have yielded mixed findings at best (i.e., some studies showed significantly slower rates while others failed to find them). The other type of evidence arises from studies of articulation rate in more real-world contexts. One long-term follow-up study suggested that children with speech sound disorders may have slower conversational articulation rates as preschoolers, though they appear to catch up to their typical speaking peers by age 12 to 16 years (Flipsen, 2002). Data from the same participants indicated that the children who failed to master a residual error (either /s/ or /r/) by their teen years did not differ significantly on conversational rate from their peers who had mastered all of the speech sounds (Flipsen, 2003). These findings suggest that while a basic assessment of speech motor skills is always a good idea, it may not provide much useful information to specifically help with remediation of /r/ errors.

Related to this is the question of oromyofunctional disorders (OMDs) and speech. There are very limited data suggesting that some children with speech sound disorders have accompanying tongue thrust or abnormal tongue resting postures. Unfortunately, no large-scale studies appear to have been carried out. A few small studies have examined whether treating OMDs may help speech (Christensen & Hanson, 1981; Overstake, 1976). Findings are difficult to interpret as they tend to show that the combination of speech treatment and OMD treatment results in the same progress for speech as doing speech treatment alone. Correcting the OMD required specific OMD treatment. Another complication is that these studies have tended to focus on /s/ errors. Published findings specific to /r/ errors appear to be lacking, so it is not clear if evaluation and/or treatment of OMDs would be of much value for assisting children with /r/ errors.

THE DIAGNOSIS

Speech sound errors may be due to perceptual problems, articulatory (motor-based) problems, or phonological problems. Some children, however, may have two or even all three of these problems at the same time. The following discussion highlights how to differentiate among these. In general, however, the child who substitutes [w] for /r/ and is stimulable for /r/ to at least the word level likely has a phonological problem. Likewise, the child whose spelling errors seem to mirror their speech errors may also have a phonological problem. The child who is not stimulable may or may not have a phonological problem but likely has an articulation problem. In general, the child who produces a distorted /r/ likely has an articulation problem. Perception should be assessed in all cases.

Assessing Stimulability

As noted, sounds that are not stimulable are assumed to represent articulatory problems. Although stimulability is defined as the speaker is able to correctly imitate a production following a model, there is actually no standard procedure for conducting this assessment. How many attempts do we make? How many different contexts should be tested? What percentage of correctly imitated productions constitutes being stimulable? Although there is no published evidence to support it being the best approach, the procedure suggested by Miccio (2002) is widely accepted. It defines being stimulable as correctly imitating a model on at least 30% of opportunities. Specifically, the child is asked to produce the sound 10 times: in isolation, and in three word positions combined with the three corner vowels (/i/, /u/, /ɑ/). The child is given three attempts to produce each of 10 targets. If the child produces any 3 or more of the 10 targets correctly even once, they are considered stimulable. Preston and Leece (2019) suggested a version of Miccio's approach, and this has been adapted in a form for conducting this assessment which is provided in Appendix 4–1.

Identifying Perceptual Problems

Having a perceptually based speech sound error means that the auditory image that is stored in long-term memory is not fully correct. It differs in some way from what other users of the language have stored in their heads. This means that when they produce the sound and they monitor their own production, they are comparing what they just said against the wrong thing. Their incorrect production may actually sound correct to them.

Over the years, several different tasks have been suggested for evaluating perceptual problems. Our friends in audiology simply read a list of words and have the person repeat the words back to them. Clearly that will not work for speech-language pathologists, because if the person says the wrong word, it is impossible to know whether they did not hear it properly or they heard it fine but just could not correctly produce the sounds.

Another very common way to test perception is using a same–different task. Typically, three pairs of words are created such as is shown below:

one-run (different)

run-one (different)

run-run (same)

one-one (same)

The first two pairs are minimal pairs that contrast the target sound with the sound the speaker typically uses in its place (the "different" pairs). The other two present no contrast between the sounds (the "same" pairs). Each of the four pairs is presented one at a time in random order. The child's task involves listening and deciding if the words are the same or different. This approach sounds like it should work. Do they notice the difference between the two sounds? However, in order to do this task, all it takes is to listen to the two words, hold them in working memory, and compare them to each other. To be successful, you only have to be able to hear the difference. Just because you are capable of hearing the difference does not mean that what is in your long-term memory is correct. The task does not require any comparison against what is in long-term memory. Therefore, it is quite possible to do this task successfully and still have a perceptual problem.

Recognizing the limitations of same–different tasks, Locke (1980) suggested that a more direct judgment task was needed. The child should be presented with correct and incorrect versions of the word (one at a time) and asked to judge whether it was produced correctly or not. The incorrect versions would be the child's error form. Doing it this way means that the child must hold the one word in their working memory and then compare it to what is in their long-term memory. There is no other way to decide. Locke called his approach the *Speech Production–Perception Task (SP-PT)*. In order to minimize misinterpretations, he created a systematic approach where a custom test is created for each child's error. Appendix 4–2 presents a form you can use for this task.

The SP-PT requires identifying three sounds, the target sound (/r/ in this context), the child's typical error (e.g., [w] or a derhotacized /r/), and a control sound. The control sound would be a similar class of sound that the child was producing correctly (/l/ can often work as a control sound for /r/; the glide /j/ could work if /l/ errors are also a problem for the child). The control sound is included to be sure the child actually understands the task. It is assumed that if the sound is being produced correctly, the child has a solid underlying representation for that sound. The SP-PT also requires presenting each of the three sounds six different times (18 total items) in random order. Including six examples of each gets around the possibility of guessing. Once identified, a stimulus item must be selected. This is one word containing the target sound. It could be represented in a picture or be a physical object. Once the word is selected, the "words to present" column is filled in on the form. A sample completed form is also included in Appendix 4–2. Using the three selected sounds, the words to present here are "ring," "wing,"[1] and "ling." A custom test for this child has now been created.

Administering the SP-PT is fairly straightforward. The clinician shows the child the stimulus picture or object and names it 18 times (one at a time) using the "word to present" column. Starting at Item 1, the clinician shows the picture and asks "is this a ling?." The child simply responds Yes or No. The clinician then circles or underlines Yes or No depending on what the child says. Then with Item 2 the clinician asks, "is this a wing?." Again, they circle or underline Yes or No depending on what the child says. Then for Item 3, they ask, "is this a ring?" and circle or underline Yes or No depending on what the child says. This is repeated for all 18 items and should take no more than a few minutes.

---

[1]If, rather than /w/, the child's error is a derhotacized /r/, that would be the error that would need to be presented to the child, not the word "wing."

Once completed, any mistakes the child made are counted. Note that on the form the correct answer is always shown in ALL CAPS. Any lower-case responses that were circled represent mistakes. Note that on the form under "Criteria," if the child makes three or more mistakes[2] when presented with the error sound, they have a perception problem. In the example, the child made five mistakes, and they were all made when their own error was presented. This suggests they thought the word "wing" was the correct way to say "ring" five out of the six times it was presented. Clearly, they were not recognizing the error—they have a perceptual problem.

Note also on the form under "Criteria" that if the child makes more than one mistake on the control sound, they may not understand the task. This is more likely to occur with very young children (under age 4 years). In such cases, Locke recommends not recording the results in the child's file but attempting the test on another day. In the example in Appendix 4–2, the child made no mistakes on either the control sound or the target sound, so we assume they understood the task.

There are at least two shortcomings to the SP-PT procedure. First, only one speaker (one voice) presents the stimuli; second, with children whose error is a derhotacized /r/, it can be very difficult to reproduce that error consistently. To get around both of these issues, an app was created called SAILS, which stands for the *Speech Assessment and Interactive Learning System*. It is available through the App Store (Rvachew & Herbay, 2017). It is based on the same basic principles as the SP-PT but contains prerecorded samples of both correct and incorrect versions of several sounds (including /r/). The samples are presented by a variety of speakers including males, females, children, and adults, which may assist with the demographic dynamics challenge discussed in Chapter 1 (i.e., mostly female vocal tract models being presented to mostly male clients). For clients who produce derhotacized /r/, the app presents multiple examples of those distortions, thus getting around the challenge of a clinician having to reproduce that error.

Like the SP-PT, the SAILS app presents the stimuli randomly. For each presentation, there is a picture of the target word on screen (target can be *rat*, *rope*, or *door* for /r/) along with a large X. The child listens to the production and then touches the picture if they believe the word was spoken correctly or the X if they believe it was a mistake. The app is designed for both assessment and perceptual training. It records performance during both modes and provides visual and auditory reinforcement during training.

Identifying Phonological Problems

As discussed earlier, regardless of the error type, a possible phonological problem must be considered. The key here is to ask whether the child

---

[2]This is *not* a norm-referenced test; it is a criterion-referenced test.

is also struggling with reading. An examination of samples of the child's spelling may also be informative. Are the spelling errors random or do they mirror what is happening in speech? Neal (2020) has suggested that if the spelling errors are similar to their speech errors, the problem may be more likely to be phonological. In addition to examining reading and spelling performance, confirmation of such problems could be made by assessment of their phonological awareness skills if this had not already been done recently. Any number of commercially available tests or informal assessments could be used. Particular attention should be paid to performance on phoneme-level tasks such as phoneme blending, phoneme segmentation, and sorting words by initial phoneme. For the child with poor performance, activities related to phonological awareness (with particular emphasis on stimuli containing /r/) can be incorporated into therapy.

ASSESSING PRODUCTION ACCURACY

Assessing accuracy of production is necessary to establish baseline performance and monitor progress toward our goals. Assuming that few ever achieve perfect accuracy all the time, a goal of 90% correct production of /r/ in conversation in all phonetic contexts seems appropriate. Although regular measurement of conversational accuracy may not be practical, for purposes of establishing a functional baseline and occasionally checking for generalization, accuracy in conversation should be measured. Using a recording of about 10 to 15 min of conversation about everyday topics, a transcript of the child's productions can be made. For most initial assessments, phonetic transcription would be needed to identify overall severity and select treatment targets. However, in cases where /r/ is the only issue, a transcript using regular spelling would be sufficient because /r/, in whatever form it appears, will always be represented in regular spelling by the letter "r." All words containing /r/ could then be underlined and specific errors circled on the transcript.

Using the transcript of the conversation as a guide, the form provided in Appendix 4–3 will allow for measurement of accuracy in singletons across the various types of /r/ from Table 2–1 as well as measurement of accuracy in /r/ initial clusters. The open squares on both parts allow for tallying each correct and incorrect instance, and then the percentage correct can be calculated for each context and each cluster along with totals for both singletons and clusters. An example of a completed scoresheet is also provided.

Generalization to nontreated words should also be explored regularly (e.g., every few weeks). The 64-item word-level probe found in McAllister Byun et al. (2014) might also prove useful for this purpose. A shorter list adapted from McAllister Byun et al. is shown in Table 4–1. The particular words in that probe would then need to be excluded from therapy

Table 4–1. Example List of Probe Words to Test for Generalization

far	root	sir	scrub	strong	rock
star	rip	her	scratch	string	green
bread	fair	trip	fruit	draw	frog
brown	pear	trash	friend	dream	train
grew	core	hammer	gear	crab	pray
grow	sore	shower	deer	crack	press

Note. Adapted from "Retroflex Versus Bunched in Treatment for Rhotic Misarticulation: Evidence From Ultrasound Biofeedback Intervention," by T. McAllister Byun, E. R. Hitchcock, and M. T. Swartz, 2014, *Journal of Speech, Language, and Hearing Research, 57*, p. 2130 (https://doi.org/10.1044/2014_JSLHR-S-14-0034).

sessions. Spontaneous productions are always preferred. If the child can read, having them read the words would suffice. For nonreaders, it may be necessary to elicit the sample via imitation.

Clinical Evidence—Tracking Progress

As discussed in Chapter 1, evidence-based practice demands that we integrate the best available published evidence with clinical expertise and client preferences and values. The published evidence shows us *what can work or what has worked elsewhere.* It does not guarantee that the approach in question will work with the client in front of us. Showing that an approach is actually working requires the ongoing collection of data as therapy is being provided. We need to show that change is happening. This is done by tracking performance on the practice items being presented in the therapy sessions (treatment data). This can simply be an ongoing tally of number of correct and incorrect attempts in the session, which is then converted to percentage values and logged.

In addition to treatment data, there is a need to show that a skill is being taught that generalizes beyond the immediate therapy sessions and therapy stimuli. In other words, are they learning anything or just performing adequately in the moment? This is done by regularly assessing performance at other linguistic levels (e.g., conversation if we are working at the word or sentence level), in other settings (e.g., on the playground or in the classroom if therapy is being done in a separate treatment room), or with other communication partners (e.g., with teachers or parents). This is generalization data, and the simplest way to gather this would be to record interactions and use the form in Appendix 4–3 to tally and estimate performance. Our ultimate goal is to have the skills we are teaching become automatic, so measuring how well the skill is generalizing to everyday speech is our strongest measure of progress.

Change happens, and we are glad when it does. However, even if change immediately follows the introduction of some therapy, it is never absolutely certain that the therapy caused the change. It may have been a coincidence, and something else may have caused the change. The child may have been on a plateau in development and then suddenly sorted something out on their own (i.e., normal development kicked in). Another possibility is that the child has been receiving therapy (formal or informal) from someone else and that additional therapy is what caused the change we are seeing. To be truly certain that the change being observed is the result of our intervention requires us to collect some control data. This involves monitoring performance on a skill that is still missing but is not being taught in therapy. These skills would be those where we would *not* expect any generalization from the therapy targets. For example, if the target is /r/ and the child also has difficulty with /s/ (and assuming no work is being done on /s/), performance on /s/ could be measured every few weeks. The idea is that if /s/ does not change, then no other factor might be influencing the outcome. If such targets are available, these should be monitored. Unfortunately, for the child whose only difficulty is with /r/, there may not be any control targets. In such cases, collecting control data may simply not be possible.

ASSESSING CONSISTENCY

Some children may have consistently poor performance across all contexts, while others may do noticeably better in particular contexts. Kent (1982) documented several sources that suggest, for example, that some children are better able to produce /r/ in particular initial clusters than in singletons. Some may do best in initial /dr/ or /tr/ clusters than in singletons. Although it is not clear why, it is likely that for these children, the tongue tip up position for the alveolar stops may encourage a retroflex action for /r/. Conversely, some children do better in initial /gr/ or /kr/ clusters. Here the raising of the dorsum of the tongue toward the velum may encourage a bunched /r/ action. Evaluating consistency, therefore, at the very beginning makes sense. The procedure used for Appendix 4–3 allows for this.

Consistency across attempts of any one particular context is also important. The conversational sample can be examined to see if words that occur more than once are consistently in error or variable. Some clients have particular words that they use often and are overlearned as either always correct or always incorrect. The former can make them appear more accurate than they really are, and the latter can make them look worse. Consistently incorrect words may need particular attention in therapy.

SUMMARY

This chapter offered our latest understanding about the assessment of persistent and residual /r/ errors and presented some procedures for doing so. In the next chapter, general treatment principles are discussed.

APPENDIX 4–1

Stimulability Probe for /r/[1]

Child's Name _____ Date _____

Target	Attempt 1	Attempt 2	Attempt 3	Number Correct	Observations
/ɝ/					
/ri/					
/iri/					
/ir/					
/rɑ/					
/ɑrɑ/					
/ɑr/					
/ru/					
/uru/					
/ur/					
Total					

Instructions:

1. Evoke each target three times in succession.

2. Provide a model before each attempt. Make the model very clear with obvious (but not exaggerated) lip rounding.

3. Instruct the child to speak slowly and make their best /r/ sound each time.

> **"Now let's say some syllables with /r/ in them. Listen and watch what I do. Then you repeat it. Take your time and try to say your very best /r/ sound."**

4. Score each attempt as correct (1) or incorrect (0). Substitutions and distortions are both considered incorrect. Note any productions that are ambiguous.

_____

[1]Adapted from Miccio (2002) and Preston and Leece (2019).

Being stimulable = 30% or greater correct (any three or more targets correct at least once).

Score (targets correct at least once): _____ / 10

Stimulable? Yes ____ No ____

APPENDIX 4–2

Speech Production–Perception Task (SP-PT) Form[1]

Child's Name _____ Date of Testing _____

Stimulus containing target sound _____

Target Sound / /   Child"s Error / /   Control Sound / /

	Word to Present		Child's Response[2]
1. Control sound in word	_____	(C)	yes NO
2. Child's error in word	_____	(E)	yes NO
3. Target sound in word	_____	(T)	YES no
4. Target sound in word	_____	(T)	YES no
5. Child's error in word	_____	(E)	yes NO
6. Control sound in word	_____	(C)	yes NO
7. Control sound in word	_____	(C)	yes NO
8. Target sound in word	_____	(T)	YES no
9. Child's error in word	_____	(E)	yes NO
10. Target sound in word	_____	(T)	YES no
11. Child's error in word	_____	(E)	yes NO
12. Control sound in word	_____	(C)	yes NO
13. Child's error in word	_____	(E)	yes NO
14. Target sound in word	_____	(T)	YES no
15. Control sound in word	_____	(C)	yes NO
16. Child's error in word	_____	(E)	yes NO
17. Target sound in word	_____	(T)	YES no
18. Control sound in word	_____	(C)	yes NO

---

[1]Adapted from Locke (1980).
[2]Correct response shown in ALL CAPS.

Number of mistakes on target sound (T):   _____

Number of mistakes on child's own error (E):   _____

Number of mistakes on control sound (C):   _____

<u>Criteria</u>:

Three or more mistakes on the child's own error = misperception (perceptual problem).

More than one mistake on control sound = child may not fully understand the task.

Interpretation: _____

_____

Instructions for Administering SP-PT

1. Identify the target phoneme and the sound the child typically uses in its place (the error). Then identify a sound that is similar to both the target and the child's error but that the child produces correctly (control). For example, if the child says "wing" for "ring," the /r/ would be the target sound, /w/ would be the child's error, and /l/ might serve as the control (assuming the child usually says /l/ correctly).

2. Under "production task," list the target word and the substitution. Using the above example:

   ring → wing

3. Write the target sound in the space marked Target ("r" in the above example), the substituted sound in the space marked Error ("w" in the above example), and the control sound in the space marked Control ("l" in the above example).

4. For each of the 18 spots under "Stimulus – Class" write the appropriate word using the sounds from Number 2 above depending on which item is listed. For example, if the item says Target, write "ring," if it says Error write "wing," and if it says Control write "ling." This creates the stimuli for the test.

5. Using the target picture as the visual cue, ask the speaker to judge whether or not you said the right word. For example:

   1. Is this "ling"?
   2. Is this "wing"?

    3. Is this "ring"?

    4. Is this "ring"?

    5. Is this "wing"? etc.

If the speaker answers "yes," underline yes next to the item. If they answer "no," underline no.

6. Where the word "yes" or "no" appears in uppercase letters, that shows the correct response. If it is in lowercase letters, that indicates it would be a mistake in perception.

7. Count up the mistakes (the number of lowercase responses) in each category (Target, Error, Control).

8. The speaker has a problem with perception if three or more mistakes in perception are noted in response to the Error stimuli. Since there are six possible Error stimuli, the child has then produced at least 50% incorrect responses. As such, it appears they are having trouble distinguishing what they usually say from what they should be saying.

9. If the child makes three or more mistakes on the Control sound, then the child may not fully understand the task. Discard results and retest at a later date.

See the following completed example.

Example SP-PT Completed Form

Child's Name _____**J. Smith**_____ Date of Testing **January 7, 2021**

Stimulus containing target sound **Picture of a ring**____

Target Sound /r/   Child's Error /w/   Control Sound /l/

	Word to Present		Child's Response[3]
1. Control sound in word	____ling____	(C)	yes **NO**
2. Child's error in word	____wing____	(E)	**yes** NO
3. Target sound in word	____ring____	(T)	**YES** no
4. Target sound in word	____ring____	(T)	**YES** no
5. Child's error in word	____wing____	(E)	**yes** NO
6. Control sound in word	____ling____	(C)	yes **NO**
7. Control sound in word	____ling____	(C)	yes **NO**
8. Target sound in word	____ring____	(T)	**YES** no
9. Child's error in word	____wing____	(E)	**yes** NO
10. Target sound in word	____ring____	(T)	**YES** no
11. Child's error in word	____wing____	(E)	**yes** NO
12. Control sound in word	____ling____	(C)	yes **NO**
13. Child's error in word	____wing____	(E)	**yes** NO
14. Target sound in word	____ring____	(T)	**YES** no
15. Control sound in word	____ling____	(C)	yes **NO**
16. Child's error in word	____wing____	(E)	yes **NO**
17. Target sound in word	____ring____	(T)	**YES** no
18. Control sound in word	____ling____	(C)	yes **NO**

Number of mistakes on target sound (T):   __5__

Number of mistakes on child's own error (E):   __0__

Number of mistakes on control sound (C):   __0__

---

[3]Child's response in bold and underlined.

<u>Criteria</u>:

Three or more mistakes on the child's own error = misperception (perceptual problem).

More than one mistake on control sound = child may not fully understand the task.

Interpretation: <u>Misperception. Child not noticing the difference between their /w/ production and the target /r/.</u>

APPENDIX 4–3

Scoresheet for Calculating /r/ Accuracy

Name _____ Date _____

Context[1]	Correct	Incorrect	% Correct
/ɝ/ initial (e.g., earth)			
/ɝ/ medial (e.g., fern)			
/ɝ/ final (e.g., fur)			
Prevocalic /r/ (e.g., red)			
/ɚ/ medial (e.g., perform)			
/rl/ medial (e.g., Charlie)			
/rl/ final (e.g., girl)			
/ɑr/ initial (e.g., art)			
/ɑr/ medial (e.g., barn)			
/ɑr/ final (e.g., car)			
/or/ initial (e.g., orange)			
/or/ medial (e.g., cork)			
/or/ final (e.g., door)			
/ir/ initial (e.g., ear)			
/ir/ medial (e.g., zero)			
/ir/ final (e.g., deer)			
/ɛr/ initial (e.g., airplane)			
/ɛr/ medial (e.g., fairy)			
/ɛr/ final (e.g., hair)			
/ɑɪr/ initial (e.g., Ireland)			
/ɑɪr/ medial (e.g., fireplace)			
/ɑɪr/ final (e.g., tire)			
SINGLETON TOTALS			

---

[1]Context list source: Ristuccia (2002).

Initial /r/ Cluster	Incorrect	% Correct	% Correct
/pr/ (e.g., prince)			
/br/ (e.g., brown)			
/tr/ (e.g., tree)			
/dr/ (e.g., dress)			
/kr/ (e.g., crown)			
/gr/ (e.g., green)			
/fr/ (e.g., frog)			
/θr/ (e.g., three)			
/spr/ (e.g., spray)			
/str/ (e.g., string)			
/skr/ (e.g., screw)			
CLUSTER TOTALS			
OVERALL TOTALS			

EXAMPLE OF COMPLETED SCORESHEET

Name ___A. B._____ Date ___1/4/2021_____

Context[2]	Correct	Incorrect	% Correct
/ɝ/ initial (e.g., earth)	lll	ₕₕₕ ₕₕₕ ₕₕₕ lll	3/21 (14%)
/ɝ/ medial (e.g., fern)		ₕₕₕ ₕₕₕ ll	0/12 (0%)
/ɝ/ final (e.g., fur)		ₕₕₕ ₕₕₕ ₕₕₕ	0/15 (0%)
Prevocalic /r/ (e.g., red)	lll	ₕₕₕ ₕₕₕ ₕₕₕ ₕₕₕ ₕₕₕ ₕₕₕ ll	3/ 35 (9%)
/ɚ/ medial (e.g., perform)	l	ₕₕₕ ₕₕₕ ₕₕₕ ₕₕₕ ₕₕₕ lll	1/29 (3%)
/rl/ medial (e.g., Charlie)		ll	0/2 (0%)
/rl/ final (e.g., girl)		ₕₕₕ ₕₕₕ	0/10 (0%)
/ɑr/ initial (e.g., art)	ll	ₕₕₕ ₕₕₕ ₕₕₕ	2/17 (12%)
/ɑr/ medial (e.g., barn)		ₕₕₕ ₕₕₕ	0/10 (0%)
/ɑr/ final (e.g., car)	l	ₕₕₕ	1/6 (17%)
/or/ initial (e.g., orange)	ll	ₕₕₕ ₕₕₕ ₕₕₕ ₕₕₕ	2/22 (9%)
/or/ medial (e.g., cork)		ₕₕₕ ₕₕₕ ₕₕₕ	0/15 (0%)
/or/ final (e.g., door)		ₕₕₕ ₕₕₕ l	0/11 (0%)
/ir/ initial (e.g., ear)	ₕₕₕ ₕₕₕ ₕₕₕ lll	ₕₕₕ ₕₕₕ ₕₕₕ	18/33 (55%)
/ir/ medial (e.g., zero)	ₕₕₕ ₕₕₕ	ₕₕₕ ₕₕₕ ₕₕₕ lll	10/28 (36%)
/ir/ final (e.g., deer)	ₕₕₕ ₕₕₕ ₕₕₕ l	ₕₕₕ ₕₕₕ ₕₕₕ ₕₕₕ ₕₕₕ ₕₕₕ	16/46 (35%)
/ɛr/ initial (e.g., airplane)	ₕₕₕ lll	ₕₕₕ ₕₕₕ ₕₕₕ ₕₕₕ ₕₕₕ ₕₕₕ llll	8/42 (19%)

---

[2]Context list source: Ristuccia (2002).

Context	Correct	Incorrect	% Correct
/ɛr/ medial (e.g., fairy)	ⵜⵜⵜ ⵜⵜⵜ	ⵜⵜⵜ ⵜⵜⵜ ⵜⵜⵜ ⵜⵜⵜ ⵜⵜⵜ lll	10/38 (26%)
/ɛr/ final (e.g., hair)	ⵜⵜⵜ ⵜⵜⵜ lll	ⵜⵜⵜ ⵜⵜⵜ ⵜⵜⵜ ⵜⵜⵜ ⵜⵜⵜ ⵜⵜⵜ ⵜⵜⵜ ⵜⵜⵜ ⵜⵜⵜ lll	13/61 (21%)
/ɑɪr/ initial (e.g., Ireland)	ll	ⵜⵜⵜ ⵜⵜⵜ ⵜⵜⵜ ⵜⵜⵜ	2/21 (9%)
/ɑɪr/ medial (e.g., fireplace)		ⵜⵜⵜ	0/4 (0%)
/ɑɪr/ final (e.g., tire)	l	ⵜⵜⵜ ⵜⵜⵜ ⵜⵜⵜ lll	1/19 (5%)
SINGLETON TOTALS	90	407	90/497 (18%)
Initial /r/ Cluster	**Correct**	**Incorrect**	**% Correct**
/pr/ (e.g., prince)		ⵜⵜⵜ ll	0/7 (0%)
/br/ (e.g., brown)		lll	0/3 (0%)
/tr/ (e.g., tree)	ⵜⵜⵜ ⵜⵜⵜ lll	ⵜⵜⵜ ll	13/20 (65%)
/dr/ (e.g., dress)	lll	ⵜⵜⵜ ⵜⵜⵜ lll	3/16 (19%)
/kr/ (e.g., crown)		llll	0/4 (0%)
/gr/ (e.g., green)	l	llll	1/5 (20%)
/fr/ (e.g., frog)		ⵜⵜⵜ lll	0/8 (0%)
/θr/ (e.g., three)		lll	0/3 (0%)
/spr/ (e.g., spray)		llll	0/4 (0%)
/str/ (e.g., string)	l	lll	1/4 (25%)
/skr/ (e.g., screw)		ll	0/2 (0%)
CLUSTER TOTALS	18	61	18/79 (23%)
OVERALL TOTALS	108	468	108/576 (19%)

CHAPTER 5

Remediation Principles

This chapter discusses general principles and suggestions related to remediation of /r/ (which could also be applied to most other speech sound targets). The goal is to set the stage for subsequent chapters that focus on specific treatment approaches.

TREAT THE ACTUAL PROBLEM

Not to state the obvious, but treatment should focus on the problem. Motor-based (articulation) treatments are the focus of most of the rest of the chapters, but given the possible co-occurring perceptual or phonological problems, some discussion for working on these is appropriate. This need not be a separate step but rather can be incorporated into motor therapy. This is followed by a discussion of some keys to making motor-based (articulation) therapy more efficient.

Perceptual Therapy

The goal of perceptual therapy is to teach the child the difference between what they are currently producing and what they should be producing or at least to bring that difference to their attention. The intent is to ensure that the child has a clear stored image in the brain of what the target is supposed to sound like. There are at least three schools of thought on doing this. The first is that such problems are so rare as to make doing this a waste of time. Although there do not appear to have been any studies of how common perceptual problems are, the lack of data at least supports the idea that we should test for it in the clients we serve. This then leads to the second school of thought, which is to test for it (as discussed in Chapter 4) and then provide perceptual therapy whenever a problem is identified. The third school of thought is that these problems are so common that we should do some type of perceptual therapy with all children with speech sound disorders. This was Van Riper's position, and it remains the position of people like Barbara Hodson who points to data on the frequency of middle ear infections in young children as the justification. Data from Shriberg (2010) indicate that up to 30% of children with speech sound disorders without any obvious cause have very frequent middle ear infections. There are also studies showing that many children experience what is called *silent otitis*, which means they have ear infections that go undetected (Marchant et al., 1984). Having a middle ear space filled with liquid can result in a moderate hearing loss. Even though it may be temporary, if this happens many times, the net result may be that the speech input the child has received has been incomplete at best or very distorted at worst. Given that this situation is so common, might it not make sense to do perceptual intervention with all children with speech sound disorders just in case? From my perspective, the most defensible position is the second school of thought. Test for it, and treat it if a problem is detected.

Relative to specific approaches to perceptual therapy, at least four different options are available. The choice of which approach to use is left up to individual clinicians at this point as there does not appear to be any published evidence suggesting that any of these options is better than any of the others.

The first option for perceptual therapy is to use the same *judgment tasks* that were suggested for assessing perception. A single item is presented (either a correct or incorrect version of a word), and the child is asked to judge whether it was produced correctly or not. They compare what they heard with what is stored in their long-term memory and decide if they match (i.e., was it correct or not?). For assessment, their responses are simply recorded, but as a therapy task, the child would immediately be told whether they had judged correctly or not. Using that corrective feedback, they would then be able to fine-tune their perception over many trials. Two specific methods for organizing and presenting these judgment tasks were mentioned in Chapter 4: the Speech Production–Perception Task approach of Locke (1980; see Chapter 4 and Appendix 4–2) and the SAILS app developed by Rvachew and Herbay (2017). Both could be used for therapy. With either approach, three to four sets of 10 trials might be presented during a treatment session, lasting perhaps 5 min in total.

A second option for perceptual therapy is the use of *same–different pairs*. Although these tasks are problematic for assessment purposes (see Chapter 4 for a discussion), they can provide the child with an opportunity to compare the target to their production form in a systematic way.

This approach would involve minimal pairs contrasting either /w/ and /r/ or a distorted /r/ and correct /r/.[1] For each contrast pair of words, there would be three pairs, such as weed-read, weed-weed, read-read. Perhaps five such contrast pairs could be created yielding 15 items to be presented. The full set of 15 would then be presented randomly. After presentation of each item, the child would have to decide if the pair was the same or different. They would then be given feedback about whether they had judged correctly or not. This would only take 2 to 3 min per treatment session. A sample set of 15 pairs for a /w/ for /r/ contrast is shown in Table 5–1. Note that for the "different" pairs the order of presentation is varied (i.e., sometimes the /r/ word is presented first, and sometimes the /w/ word is presented first). This is done to prevent the child from guessing and (more importantly) to force the child to focus on the acoustic details of both words.

A third option for perceptual training could be termed *discrimination drill*. Here word pairs contrasting /w/ and /r/ could be presented orally along with accompanying pairs of pictures. The clinician would say one of the words, and the child would be required to point to the correct picture. In later sessions, the task could be made more challenging by presenting groups of pictures that represent several different contrast pairs all at once. One word would be presented orally, and the child would have to identify the correct picture from among the larger set.

Table 5–1. Example of Contrast Pair Activity List for Same–Different Perceptual Therapy

Word Pair	Status	Word Pair	Status
walk-walk	Same	ring-wing	Different
ride-wide	Different	walk-rock	Different
run-run	Same	one-one	Same
ride-ride	Same	right-right	Same
run-one	Different	white-right	Different
white-white	Same	rock-rock	Same
ring-ring	Same	wing-wing	Same
wide-wide	Same		

---

[1]If the contrast is with a distortion, it might be useful to prerecord all of the pairs to be presented to ensure some consistency in presentation. It can be challenging for most of us to consistently reproduce a distorted /r/.

Any of these tasks could be done either at the beginning or the end of a therapy session to accompany production activities. Intuitively, doing it at the beginning may be slightly more useful (although there is no specific evidence supporting this) as it may help focus the child's attention and set the stage for production practice.

The notion of doing both perceptual and production therapy together in the same session is inherent in the fourth option for perceptual therapy. This involves a form of intensive modeling which Barbara Hodson (2010) refers to as *amplified auditory stimulation* (some mistakenly call this auditory bombardment which is not a term Hodson uses). In this case, at both the beginning and end of the therapy session (with production practice activities in between), the clinician reads lists of words containing the target sound (no particular number of words is specified, but 30 to 50 seems reasonable). Hodson strongly suggests that the word lists be read through some sort of amplification system (e.g., Pocket Talker). This ensures the productions are clear and avoids the tendency to distort the signal that occurs for all of us when trying to talk louder. In terms of how to read the lists, Hodson has suggested two possible approaches. First, the words could simply be read with about a 1-s pause between each word. Alternatively, the words could each be read along with the child's error (e.g., read–weed, one–run). Another option, which I have used, is to present three words for each item: correct version, child's version, correct version again (e.g., "ride-wide-ride"[2]). The logic of this latter format is to present a contrast but provide two models of the correct form to help the child focus more heavily on that version. Regardless of the format of presentation, the child need not do anything while the words are being read. They only listen. The listening session would not take more than 4 to 6 min (2 to 3 min each at the beginning and end) out of any one treatment session. Table 5–2 provides an example of a word list that could be used for initial /r/.

Phonological Therapy

The overall goal of speech sound intervention is to create and/or solidify what is stored in long-term memory about specific speech sounds. As noted previously, consistently correct production requires a strong association between what the target sounds like, what it feels like, and how it functions in the language. Phonological intervention puts a heavy emphasis on teaching the child about the function of the sound in the language (i.e., how it generates and contrasts meaning).

---

[2]If the child's error is a distortion, that would be presented as the middle item. As with the same–different pairs approach, these might be prerecorded to ensure consistency of presentation.

Table 5–2. Example of Listening List That Could Be Used with Amplified Auditory Stimulation for /r/ Initial

race	rack	rave	rig
ram	raw	rich	ride
rise	ray	rat	rim
risk	raft	roam	ripe
reel	robe	rink	rid
rinse	rent	rice	rack
reef	rake	rock	rind
rain	rags	ramp	rip
road	roast	read	rover
right	reap	write	red

Phonological production therapy would be appropriate for the child who substitutes [w] for /r/ if they are also stimulable for /r/ to the word level. It would also be appropriate for the same child who was not previously stimulable but who has progressed to the word level with articulation therapy. In other words, if they have been substituting [w] for /r/, production practice at the word level and above should involve a phonological approach. At least two different types of activities could be used for this (see later). Minimal pairs may also be presented (regardless of stimulability) early in therapy to demonstrate to the child how using different sounds results in different meaning.

Minimal Pairs Production Practice

The most well-established form of phonological therapy (and the one with the most supporting evidence) is known as minimal pairs therapy. The basic idea is to create a series of minimal pairs that contrast /w/ and /r/ (see the "different" pairs in Table 5–1 for some examples). After discussing the meanings of the words being used, these can be presented in any number of drill or game activities with pictures illustrating each word. The child is required to correctly produce all the words, with /w/ or /r/ as appropriate. Feedback is provided about correctness so the child develops a strong sense of a correct /w/ production versus a correct /r/ production.

Beyond the word level, the activities can be made more challenging by requiring production of the word in a structured phrase during the production activity. Examples include "I see a _____" or "That is a _____" or "This card shows a picture of _____." A next step might be to have the child generate a unique sentence for each word that would be written on the picture. The child would then have to produce those unique sentences during the drill or game activity.

Phonological Awareness Activities

The second type of phonological therapy activities include those that are most appropriate for any child who is also struggling with reading and writing (regardless of their error type). These should focus on the phoneme level (see Melby-Lervag et al., 2012, for a discussion). The following are some possible activities. Note that rhyming is not included here as there is little evidence that it helps much. Note also that the picture cards being used would *not* have anything written on them to avoid the child simply looking for the written letter. Later activities might include the written form on the pictures and could assist with teaching letter-sound correspondences that may be happening in early grade classrooms.

Phoneme sorting tasks would require the child to sort out a random set of cards containing both /r/ and /w/. The cards can be reviewed initially to make sure the child knows the words. Two different levels of this task can be used. Initially the clinician would say the words one at a time and ask the child to decide which sound the word started with and then put it into a pile for that sound. All the words could then be sorted. The next level of this task would be to spread out all the pictures and have the child sort them without the clinician saying anything. The child would say the words out loud as they put them into the appropriate piles.

Phoneme segmentation tasks require the child to sound out each word. Words containing both /w/ and /r/ would be mixed together. Then the task can be modeled. "This word is 'run.' The sounds in this word are /r/, /ʌ/, and /n/." They are then asked to do the same with the rest of the words, one at a time.

Phoneme blending tasks require the child to listen to a segmented word and then merge the sounds together to create the word. For example, "Let's put sounds together into words. If I say the sounds /r/, /ʌ/, and /n/, what word does it make?" After doing the words one at a time, the task can be elevated by laying out in front of the child several contrasting pairs of picture cards for the words being practiced. The instructions then become something like, "If I say the sounds /r/, /ʌ/, and /n/, which picture does that word go with?" The child then picks out the picture that goes with the word. It can be made even more challenging by laying out all of the pictures at once and then presenting the segmented words one at a time.

It is worth noting that, as with perceptual therapy activities, by themselves, phonological awareness activities are unlikely to improve production. These would need to at least be conducted alongside production activities. For the child with multiple error sounds, a combined program such as Metaphon (see Hesketh, 2010) may also be worth considering.

ARTICULATION THERAPY AND
PRINCIPLES OF MOTOR LEARNING

As noted, a good deal of our efforts at remediating residual or persistent /r/ errors will be about improving articulatory or speech motor skill. Speech is a complex motor task. One suggested reason for our lack of success with remediating this sound is that our approach to this most complex motor task has not been sufficiently systematic. We can probably learn a lot from our colleagues in fields such as physical therapy and kinesiology who have studied this in much more detail and now speak of motor learning principles. These principles can provide a more structured framework for our work. Although many of the points that follow may not be new to most readers, our field has only recently begun to frame them in this way.

Before discussing specific principles of motor learning, it is important to recall the overall goal. Imagine the first time you tried a new motor task such as playing golf or knitting or hanging wallpaper. As you tried it the first time, you likely began in a very slow and deliberate way. As the movements slowly became more familiar, you started to make the connection between the movements and the goal being targeted, and the task became easier. Those connections were strengthened by the feedback you received from your motor and sensory systems (auditory, tactile, proprioceptive, kinesthetic) as well as the feedback you received from others. Ultimately, if you stuck with it long enough, the skill became almost automatic (i.e., you did it without much thought). At that point, you were able to quickly and flexibly adapt the basic movement patterns (motor plans) that you had learned to the changing demands of varying circumstances. If you have learned to knit and have practiced it a lot, knitting a sweater with very coarse wool is now probably not any more difficult than knitting a pair of gloves with very fine wool. That automaticity and flexibility is the goal of learning for any motor task.

Flexibility in speech means being able to adapt to the varying phonetic combinations of different words, the varying grammatical combinations of different sentence structures, and the varying emotional (prosodic) demands of the situation. Almost every speech act is unique; we have never produced it before. As a result, it is not possible to memorize all of the possible variations that might be encountered, so developing the flexibility to adapt is essential. Therapy then needs to be structured so as to teach a flexible skill, not the memorization of a set of prepackaged forms. Following the principles of motor learning should allow us to teach that flexibility and build up to that automaticity.

Discussions of the underlying principles of motor learning are typically organized in terms of principles related to setting up the learning or prepractice, the practice itself, the focus of attention during practice, and the way in which feedback is provided. Much of what follows was taken from Maas and colleagues (2008) and Schmidt and Lee (2005).

Prepractice Goals

Prior to actually beginning any therapy, the conditions for possible success should be maximized. This is done by targeting a least two broad goals. First, we want to ensure there is enough motivation for learning to take place. This is accomplished by making sure the client understands what we are attempting to do and why. Explaining the overall goal and how we hope to get there is crucial to this. We cannot simply assume that parents or teachers have already done this. It may also include discussing with the client any negative impacts they may be experiencing. Likewise, it can be helpful to discuss the specific therapy activities and perhaps offer them choices.

The second prepractice goal is to ensure task understanding. The instructions need to be clear and age appropriate, and there should be no ambiguity about what sort of responses are considered correct or not. In the case of /r/, this includes the clinician being able to make consistent judgments about what is a distortion versus a substitution versus a correct production so that consistent feedback can be provided (see discussion on transcribing and scoring productions in Chapter 4). Related to this is ensuring that the child is able to process the information presented during the task. If they are supposed to be wearing glasses or hearing aids, these should be present, functioning, and in use.

Practice Principles

Practice Amount (Dosage or Intensity)

There are several principles related to actual practice to consider when trying to optimize outcomes for learning any new motor skill. The first of these relates to treatment dosage or how much practice is needed. Not surprisingly, the research suggests that more practice is generally better. A review by Hitchcock, Swartz, and Lopez (2019a), for example, suggested a small but significant relationship between treatment intensity (number of trials per session combined with the number of sessions) and treatment success. More practice provides more chances to build the associations among the way the target sounds, the way it feels, and the meaning it signals. It also provides more opportunities to retrieve the basic motor plans leading to faster development of automaticity. There are at least two caveats on possible dosage. First, any perceptual therapy included in a treatment session (where necessary) may limit the amount of time spent in production practice. Second, it is likely that in early sessions, orientation to tasks and procedures may also limit practice trials somewhat. It should still, however, be possible to do many trials in a session.

It is not yet clear what the optimal production dose should be, but three reviews offer some insight. Williams (2012) reviewed four treatment studies in detail and suggested a minimum of at least 50 trials per 30-min treatment session was necessary for treatment success. Sugden and colleagues (2018) reviewed almost 200 treatment studies and observed that "(w)hen it was reported, the most common dose was 100 production trials within a 30–45 minute session" (p. 724). Preston, Leece, and Storto (2019) reviewed six treatment studies that used an approach called speech motor chaining (discussed later) and found that the participants were able to attempt an average of 218 trials in treatment sessions lasting up to 52 min. Together, this suggests a goal of up to 100 production trials per 30-min session is not an unreasonable expectation. This amounts to only three trials per minute, which is slightly less than the approximately 3.5 trials per minute that Skelton and Hagopian (2014) reported achieving in their study with three 4- to 6-year-old children.

Practice Distribution

A second practice principle is related to dosage. It is the question of how practice is distributed over time. Massed practice involves many trials over a short period of time (i.e., relatively fewer but longer sessions), while distributed practice spreads the trials over a longer period (i.e., many shorter sessions). Limited evidence is available to demonstrate whether either approach yields better outcomes. A 2019 study by Maas and colleagues involving six children with childhood apraxia suggested that massed practice results in "more robust motor learning," although data from at least two children failed to support that conclusion.

Practice Variability

A third practice principle is the question of whether constant practice of a single stimulus is better than variable practice involving many different stimuli. Maas et al. (2008) reviewed the very limited evidence related to speech skill in this area and concluded that neither is absolutely better than the other. However, they suggested that practicing only a single stimulus *may* be of more benefit early in therapy, while variable practice with multiple stimuli later in therapy may be more valuable. The discussion from Chapter 2 regarding different kinds of /r/ may be relevant here. Given the complexity of /r/, it may be that focusing on specific /r/ forms (see Table 2–1) might be worth trying in the early stages of therapy. As therapy progresses, however, the different forms should likely be integrated into the same therapy activities to ensure flexibility.

Practice Schedule

In instances where multiple stimuli are being practiced, another principle to be addressed is how practice should be scheduled. Should the stimuli be practiced on a blocked or random basis? For example, if there are 20 stimuli and the goal is 100 total trials, each stimulus could be practiced five times in a row followed by five trials of the next stimuli and so on (blocked practice), or the 20 stimuli could be practiced in random order once each and this could then be repeated five times (random practice). Results from a study by Geertsema and le Roux (2019) suggested no clear advantage for either schedule. Wong and colleagues in 2013 reported a similar general conclusion but included a combined condition. Findings indicated that a mix of blocked and random presentation may be the most beneficial. It did not appear to matter whether the blocked or random practice occurred first. On the other hand, a study by Adams and Page (2000) suggested superior results for a random schedule.

Part Versus Whole Practice

A final practice principle relates to how much of the task should be practiced. In this case, the question is whether speech should be broken down into its parts or practiced as a whole motor act. As far back as 1931, Travis addressed this question by stating "a sound is the very smallest possible unit with which to deal. It should not be broken up into the movements out of which one might suppose it to be built" (p. 228). Travis did not provide any evidence to support this position, and evidence on the part versus whole question continues to be lacking relative to speech. However, studies of complex, nonspeech motor activities suggest that practicing the whole act is of much greater value. Speech is, by definition, a complex motor act. From a practical perspective, performing the whole task makes more intuitive sense than just doing parts of it. Imagine learning to play golf where the most important skill you have to learn is how to swing the club. The golf instructor will tell you things like how to grip the club, how to position your feet, how to turn your hips and your shoulders, and how to hold your head. After demonstrating to you each of these things, the instructor will ask you to swing the club (i.e., to perform the entire task). They will not have you grip and release the club dozens of times in a row or position your feet dozens of times in a row. With complex tasks like this, the only way to truly learn it is to do the whole task. Speech is an equally complex task—in fact, some have described speech as the single most gymnastic activity human beings ever engage in (with all due respect to gymnasts). It makes sense, therefore, to do the whole task in order to learn to do it properly. In other words, therapy activities should include production of at least a complete speech sound and perhaps even a complete syllable.

Focus of Attention

During speech therapy activities, it is possible for the client to focus their attention on either the pattern of movements by the articulators (i.e., what did it feel like?) or the acoustic result of those movements (i.e., was that a good /r/?). Focusing on the individual movements is usually described as having an *internal* focus, while focusing on the acoustic output is described as having an *external* focus. Some studies of non-speech motor skills have suggested an external focus may be superior. However, little study of speech motor skills and attention appears to have been conducted. In 2016, McAllister Byun and colleagues looked at this question in a study of visual acoustic feedback for /r/ with nine children aged 6;8 to 13;3. Six of the nine children showed improved performance on at least one version of /r/ in 8 weeks of therapy, but the type of focus did not significantly predict outcomes. The authors noted that by its very nature, visual acoustic feedback tends to direct the child's attention to the movement of the articulators (an internal focus). Therefore, it is not clear whether either type of focus might be best for interventions that do not provide visual feedback (i.e., the types of interventions most clinicians currently use).

Given our limited knowledge on this question, it makes sense to experiment with each client to see what might work for them in terms of where to focus their attention. Alternatively, you might consider a suggestion that currently has no supporting empirical evidence. Perhaps early on when learning a brand new skill, such as how to produce a good /r/ in isolation, it makes sense to focus on the movements of the articulators. Once that /r/ is established (or if the child is already stimulable for /r/), it might make sense to quickly switch to focusing on the sound being produced (i.e., was that a good /r/?). Using the feedback principles described later in this chapter, this allows the child to take charge of their own improvement. Given all of the possible ways in which speakers can produce a good /r/ (recall our discussion in Chapter 2), they can adjust whatever they need to using the feedback from their own systems combined with whatever feedback we provide. It also encourages self-monitoring, which is discussed later.

Feedback Principles

Once a client attempts a skill we are trying to teach them, we give them feedback so they can learn from what just happened. Four aspects of that feedback deserve our attention. The first two relate to the kind of information we provide to the client. First there is the *general feedback type*. We can give information about the specific things they did which are correct or incorrect (knowledge of performance [KP]). This is often specific to the particular target sound (i.e., focusing on specific articulators or places in the vocal tract). Alternatively, we can provide our clients with information about whether or not they produced the right result (knowledge of results [KR]). This is typically more generic feedback. Some examples of the two types of feedback are shown in Table 5–3. Note that some of the examples assume that visual feedback like electropalatography (EPG) or ultrasound is available, which may not be true in all cases.

The available research is limited but suggests that KP is valuable in the early stages of therapy when the client is still not sure about the move-

Table 5–3. Examples of Different Kinds of Feedback

Positive Feedback	Negative Feedback
Knowledge of Performance (KP) for /r/	
[retroflex /r/]	[retroflex /r/]
Good, your tongue tip was raised.	No, not quite. Lift up the front of your tongue a bit.
[retroflex /r/]	[retroflex /r/]
Yes, the back of your tongue was down.	Not quite. Keep the back of your tongue down.
[bunched /r/]	[bunched /r/]
Got it! The sides of your tongue were up.	No. Lift the sides of your tongue up.
[bunched /r/]	[bunched /r/]
Good, your tongue tip was down.	Not quite right. Remember to keep your tongue tip down.
[any form of /r/]	[any form of /r/]
Yes, you kept your lips steady.	No, your lips were sticking out too much.
Knowledge of Results (KR)—Generic	
Correct.	Not that one.
Excellent!	Not quite.
Way to go!	No, not that time.
Good one.	No.
Great.	Didn't get that one.

Note. Adapted from "Tutorial: Speech Motor Chaining Treatment for School-Age Children With Speech Sound Disorders," by J. L. Preston, M. C. Leece, and J. Storto, 2019, *Language, Speech, and Hearing Services in Schools*, 50, p. 348 (https://doi.org/10.1044/2018_LSHSS-18-0081).

ment pattern (i.e., when they do not yet have an internal model of what the movement is supposed to feel like). KR may be more useful later in therapy, once the behavior is established and our goal becomes promoting generalization and automaticity. It is thought that KR may allow the client to evaluate their own errors and take control of their own learning by combining the KR with their own internal feedback.

A third aspect of feedback is *feedback quantity* or how much to provide. Whether we provide KP or KR, should we comment on every trial, every other trial, or every few trials? There is again limited research on this question. Some early studies have suggested that high-frequency feedback may assist performance on individual trials but may inhibit long-term learning. One possible explanation is that learners who receive a lot of feedback come to rely too heavily on the feedback and fail to use their own internal feedback for learning (see Wulf & Shea, 2004, for a discussion). A few studies provide some relevant data. Steinberg Lowe and Buchwald (2017) studied 32 normal adults during the learning of nonwords. They compared feedback on 100%, 50%, 20%, and 0% of trials, and findings suggested that feedback on 50% of trials provided the best outcomes. Another study of 40 normal adults by Adams and Page (2000) involved teaching them to produce a standard phrase at about half of the normal speaking rate. Retention of the skill 2 days later proved to be much better for those who received feedback every fifth trial (20% rate) compared to those who received feedback after every trial. Maas, Butalla, and Farinella (2012) studied four children with childhood apraxia of speech comparing 100% and 60% feedback conditions and reported mixed results. Two children showed better results from the 60% condition; findings for the other two could not be easily interpreted because of other confounding influences. Finally, Kim, LaPointe, and Stierwalt (2012) looked at the combination of both feedback frequency and amount of practice in 32 English-speaking adults attempting to learn to pronounce words in Korean. Specifically, they compared combinations of either 25 or 100 trials with either 100% feedback or 20% feedback. They reported that best results were obtained with 100 trials and 20% feedback. It should be noted that these studies each looked at a fixed frequency of feedback. If high-frequency feedback assists with learning in individual trials, perhaps it is most useful in the early stages of therapy. Rather than setting a fixed rate of feedback, an alternative might be to begin with high-frequency feedback to maximize information available but reduce the frequency as therapy progresses. This then might encourage automaticity, as it would allow the client to come to rely mostly on their own internal feedback. This is a core component of the speech motor chaining approach (to be discussed later) by Preston, Leece, and Storto (2019).

A final aspect of feedback relates to *feedback timing* or when the feedback should be provided. Should it be provided immediately after the trial, or should there be a delay? The available literature is once again limited but tends to suggest that a delay of up to 5 s yields better outcomes. Delaying the feedback gives the client an opportunity to experience and process their own feedback and thus take charge of their own learning.

Box 5–1: Summary of Motor Learning Principles

1. Ensure motivation: provide clear goals with clear justification

2. Ensure task understanding: make sure instructions and expectations are clear

3. Ensure task understanding: make sure sensory systems (hearing, sight) are functional

4. More practice is better: try for at least 100 production trials per 30 min

5. Fewer longer sessions *may* be better than many shorter sessions

6. Use focused drills on a few stimuli very early and more and varied stimuli as treatment progresses

7. Use a mix of blocked and random practice

8. Practice the whole task rather than individual parts

9. Focus on either movements or output (*may* vary by client) (*perhaps* focus on movements early; switch to focus on output once target established)

10. Provide KP early, but switch to KR once behavior is established

11. Begin with lots of feedback but decrease amount over time

12. Wait up to 5 s before providing feedback

Implementing the Principles of Motor Learning

In most discussions of traditional articulation therapy, the idea of task difficulty is usually framed in terms of linguistic levels (i.e., isolation, syllables, words, phrases, sentences, conversation). However, the discussion of motor learning principles suggests that there is much more involved. Coordinating all of these elements would appear to be a considerable challenge.

Fortunately, a review of Box 5–1 suggests that most of these principles only need to be considered once and would not likely vary during therapy for any particular child. This includes the prepractice principles (Items 1 to 3) and the notion that more is better (Item 4). It also includes Item 5, as for most school-based clinicians, session length is either predetermined by school or district policy or is limited by available time in their schedules. Practicing the whole speech movement (Item 8) and delaying feedback (Item 12) also need not change as therapy progresses.

However, the net result is that following motor learning principles would still require the coordination of at least five of the principles (Items 6, 7, 9, 10, 11). This is not a small challenge and suggests the need for some sort of systematic approach to avoid losing track. A checklist to assist with this is shown in Appendix 5–1. Note that it also includes space for tracking progress. A partially completed hypothetical example is also included to illustrate its use.

An alternative for keeping track of the process is built into an approach proposed by Preston, Leece, and Storto (2019) called *speech motor chaining* (SMC).[3] For this approach, a chain is a sequence of progressively longer stimuli (syllable, monosyllabic word, multisyllabic word, phrase, self-generated sentence). Each chain includes a specific phoneme combination. The initial chain is selected because of some facilitating context (see Chapter 6), and at the multisyllabic level, the target sound is placed in a stressed syllable. Once a particular chain is mastered, a related chain is then practiced. Once a particular context is mastered, another context is introduced and practiced. Despite the fact that there may be 21 different contexts for /r/ (see Table 2–1), it is unlikely that all 21 contexts would need to be practiced. Regular probing of conversation (see Appendix 4–3) would allow for monitoring of generalization to the other contexts.

Three possible chain examples for word initial /r/ include the following:

/rɪ/ – rib – ribbon—a blue ribbon [self-generated, e.g., "He won a blue ribbon."]

/ri/ – read – reading—reading a good book [self-generated, e.g., "He is reading a good book today."]

/gre/ – great – grateful—grateful for the help [self-generated, e.g., "I'm so grateful for the help."]

Note that for purposes of SMC, production of the sound in isolation is considered to be "prepractice," where the sound is evoked using typical placement, shaping, and/or other cuing. Possible cues for evoking /r/ are discussed in the next chapter. The cues that are found to be helpful for the

---

[3]The authors of this approach do not claim it accounts for all of the Principles of Motor Learning, but it does account for many of them. There are several studies supporting its overall efficacy.

child are noted and can be used as reminders if the child has difficulty at higher levels in the chain. Once at least three correct productions of the sound in isolation are achieved, the chain is begun at the syllable level. The child is then asked to attempt the syllable target a total of six times. Different kinds of feedback are presented (KP, KR; randomly) for most trials, and each production is scored as correct or incorrect. The child is also required to judge the correctness of their last three attempts. If the child produces five of six attempts correctly, they move up to the next level in the chain (this translates to 83% correct and is consistent with the Challenge Point framework discussed later). If they have fewer than five correct, they are asked to attempt the syllable one more time. If they achieve five of six correct, they then move up to the next level in the chain. If they are unsuccessful on the second attempt at any level, or if they are successful at all levels of a chain, a new chain with a new syllable is introduced.

In addition to practicing each stimulus, at the monosyllabic level and above, prosodic variations are introduced randomly. For example, the child may be asked to say the target at a slow or fast pace, or as a question rather than a statement, or to say it loudly or softly. As they progress up the levels of the chain, less and less feedback is provided. While this sounds rather complicated, a scoring form that incorporates all of this is provided in the Preston, Leece, and Storto (2019) paper. A free version of the paper is available at https://osf.io/5jmf9/. That same site includes a fillable online form so that the stimuli and feedback can be customized to each child. Also included is a video tutorial for using the form and the approach.

MAKING PROGRESS IN THERAPY—THE CHALLENGE POINT

Regardless of the particular therapy approach being used, there will usually be a series of steps involved to move the client from where they currently are to achievement of the final goal. What determines when to move from one step to the next? Until recently, there has been little guidance for the individual clinician. I can recall struggling with this issue myself. How can I be sure that the child has mastered that particular skill level and is ready for the next one? In occasional discussions with clinicians, this appears to be a common problem. My very subjective sense is that many of us are spending too much time on any one particular level in therapy.

The relatively new concept of the "challenge point," which appears to be quite similar to Vygotsky's zone of proximal development, may help in this regard. The idea is to maximize learning by making the task just hard enough to avoid both boredom and frustration. That is, we present tasks that are not too easy, not too hard, but just right (what some have called being in the Goldilocks Zone).

What we are really talking about here is making therapy as efficient as possible. Hitchcock, Swartz, and Lopez (2019b) noted that if the task is too easy and accuracy is high, the child is not receiving any meaningful feedback, and there is little opportunity for them to learn anything. If this situation persists, they may easily become bored. But if the task is too difficult and accuracy is low, they may become overwhelmed by too much negative feedback and be unable to learn from it. This may result in the child becoming frustrated. Some sweet spot in the middle needs to be found so that they get enough positive feedback to be encouraged to keep trying but enough negative feedback to be challenged to improve. Hence, it is called the *challenge point*. Exactly where that point might be is still somewhat unclear, but so far it looks like it should be somewhere between 50% and 80% correct. If the child is performing above 80%, the task is too easy. If they are performing at below 50%, the task is too hard. By monitoring performance on treatment stimuli, this framework provides a structure for how to progress in therapy:

performance below 50% correct: make the task easier

performance above 80% correct: make the task harder

performance at 50% to 80% correct: continue practice at that level

Making the task easier or harder would involve modifying one or more of the elements tracked in Appendix 5–1 (linguistic level, number of stimuli, blocked or random practice, focus of attention, KP or KR feedback, feedback frequency). The example in Appendix 5–1 illustrates this. Performance on 3/16/20 was 80% correct. However, it was based on practicing only four word stimuli in blocked practice, and feedback was provided on 80% of trials. For the next session (3/18/20), the number of stimuli was increased to 16 words, random practice was introduced, and feedback was reduced to 25% of trials. Despite all these changes, the child was 89% correct, which justified moving to the phrase level at the next session. The number of elements changed at any one time could vary by the client and how they respond. In particular, if their progress drops sharply when more than one element is changed, the number of changed elements can be reduced (effectively making the task easier).

GENERALIZATION BEYOND THE THERAPY ROOM

Children typically spend much more time outside of therapy practicing their errors than they do in therapy correcting them. How do we ensure that what they are learning in therapy will transfer to the rest of their communication? This issue may be even more of a challenge for children with persistent errors than those with residual errors. Recall from Chapter 3 that children with persistent errors would have been producing a distorted /r/ from a very early age and would have strongly ingrained habits. Contrast that with children with residual errors who would have been producing [w] for /r/ substitutions for a good deal of time before they transitioned to a distortion error. As such, they would have spent less time practicing those distortions.

Regardless of the origin of the errors, generalization is a significant concern. Some children appear to generalize quite easily from one situation to another, but this is not true for most of those we serve. Unfortunately, the studies that have attempted to identify the factors that facilitate generalization have yielded very mixed results. Lacking clear guidance, the safest approach to generalization would be to take a systematic approach.

Some of what has already been discussed in this chapter actually represents part of that planning. By following the principles of motor learning, generalization is being built into the process. The child is being encouraged to take charge of their own improvement. By shifting from providing mostly knowledge of performance to knowledge of results, fading out feedback, and delaying that feedback when we do provide it all encourages the child to pay attention to the feedback they receive from their own systems. This builds automaticity that we hope will be the basis for generalization. The self-evaluation of correctness and the self-generation of the sentence-level stimuli included in the previously discussed speech motor chaining approach (Preston, Leece, & Storto, 2019) are also examples of trying to build in the potential for automaticity.

As any experienced clinician will tell you, however, automaticity in the therapy room is one thing, but automaticity in other settings may be something else entirely. Many clinicians can cite examples of children who produce beautifully clear and highly consistent target productions in the therapy room but show little generalization outside the room. I can recall the case of a young boy who was performing wonderfully in the therapy session (85% accuracy that day). However, when the session ended, he took two steps outside the door, turned to a school staff member, and immediately returned to producing his error pattern. I was standing only 3 feet away. Talk about bursting your bubble.

So why does generalization fail to occur? The behavior may simply not yet be fully solidified, and more practice may be needed. Another possibility is that it is the result of what psychologists refer to as *state dependent learning*. This is where "information acquired in a certain state requires a similar state for best recall" (Radulovic et al., 2017, p. 92). The state likely includes any or all of the physical and sensory conditions that were present during learning (conditions that might include you as a clinician and the room you are working in). If those conditions change, it may result in those memories not being recalled. This may be especially true when stored memories for the same or similar activities are already associated in the brain with a different set of conditions (i.e., a different behavioral habit is linked to that other set of conditions). This might be why ingrained bad habits become difficult to overcome. The new behavior needs to become more strongly associated with those different conditions. This supports the idea that generalization requires specific planning.

For many readers, much of what follows here is not especially new. Many of these elements have been discussed for years. Given that the empirical evidence for any or all of these is largely lacking, applying them systematically still represents our best hope to encourage generalization.

Measure It

Without actually measuring it, there is no sure way to know whether generalization is happening. Asking teachers and parents whether they are noticing changes in the child's speech is helpful, but it is not sufficient. They are in the same situation as all other typical listeners. They are mostly interested in whether the message can be understood. More importantly, they are not taking systematic samples of the child's speech. That is our role. Visiting the child in different circumstances (e.g., the classroom, the playground, the lunchroom) or calling them at home is the only way to know for sure if generalization is happening. We can record 5 to 10 min of conversation and evaluate it using the scoresheet in Appendix 4–3. Taking a generalization sample at least once a month should be sufficient.

Incorporate Self-Assessment and Self-Monitoring

As noted previously, encouraging automaticity within the therapy session is part of the process of encouraging generalization. We can start with teaching self-assessment. As the child approaches 50% accuracy at the word level, we can ask the child whether they think their production was correct or not. Then we can tell them what we think (i.e., provide the feedback).

Self-monitoring is a variation on self-assessment in that it involves keeping track of your own spontaneous productions. We can teach them to pay attention by starting with ourselves. We can start by reading sentences aloud. Ask them to simply raise a finger every time they hear the /r/ sound. This can be expanded to short paragraphs. Then we can show them pictures and ask them to make up sentences about them. We will then raise our finger whenever we hear the /r/ sound. Once they get the idea, they need to identify the /r/ sounds in their own sentences. This can progress to be a short activity involving 3 to 5 min of conversation to end each session where they are identifying all of the /r/ sounds in both their and your speech.

Where parents are willing and able, you can incorporate them into the process. You can send home short paragraphs for them to read to the child who then has to listen and identify all of the /r/ sounds being produced. By the way, did you notice the 10 /r/ sounds in the last two sentences?

Incorporate Self-Generated Stimuli

The speech motor chaining approach discussed previously requires that the last level of the chain be a short sentence generated by the child that includes the phrase they just practiced. This can be incorporated into any approach. Take the picture stimuli you are using, and have the child generate a sentence for each of those words. These can be practiced as sentence-level stimuli. You can also photocopy that list of sentences and send it home with the child to practice as homework.

Using self-generated stimuli does several things. First, it makes what is being practiced more meaningful to the child. They decided what to say which reinforces its importance. Second, and related to the first, is that, when these are sent home, the child can have a sense of ownership or pride in that they designed their own homework. Third, it requires them to generate unique motor programs for the utterances, and thus reinforces motor planning skill. Finally, it adds to the variety of stimuli being practiced, which we know is important from the principles of motor learning.

Practice and Measure in Conversation

The ultimate goal of our work on speech is its correct use in everyday conversation. Assuming that the new behavior will automatically happen at this level without actually practicing and measuring at this level makes no sense. Engaging the child in conversation within the therapy sessions (and checking their accuracy while doing it) should be part of the generalization process. This can be done every few weeks.

Change the Setting

Associating the new behavior with the new state means actually practicing the new behavior under a different set of conditions. On a regular basis, therefore, you should try to do the therapy session in different places. These other places could be the library, an unoccupied classroom, the gym, the lunchroom, or (weather permitting) out on the playground.

Another possibility would be (assuming in-person sessions are the norm) to do occasional sessions via telepractice. This will expand the set of conditions (environmental cues) that the child is associating with the new speech behavior.

Add Homework

No one likes giving homework, and no one likes doing homework. However, having the new correct /r/ productions practiced at home may be crucial to seeing generalization. It allows for the association of the new speech behavior with a whole new set of conditions.

Some parents are very willing and eager to help. Stephen Sacks (2020, personal communication) suggests that most are likely to help to some extent under three conditions: (a) you make it clear why it will help their child's speech, (b) you are clear about what you expect them to do and how they should respond to their child, and (c) you do not ask too much. For most parents, 5 min of work each weeknight should be doable. Clearly there will be situations where homework is not practical or parents are not willing to help. All we can do, however, is ask. Assuming they agree, we can ask them to fill out a log showing that the homework was done.

Homework is probably not a good idea until the child is working at the word level and producing a relatively high level of accuracy. At that point, you can discuss homework with the parents and (assuming they are willing) begin sending home copies of the practice stimuli at one level below the one that the child is currently working on (this ensures practice of correct productions). As they become comfortable with that, you can also add in the /r/ identification discussed earlier. Once the child reaches the sentence level, you can replace the word practice with practice of the self-generated sentences.

In terms of how much time parents should spend with their child doing speech homework, there is no clear answer to this question. Clearly the more that is done the better, but asking for too much may only lead to parents getting frustrated if they cannot do as much as we ask. This may lead to them giving up on homework and not doing any. Stephen Sacks (2020, personal communication) observed that young clinicians tend to ask for a lot, but that many come to realize over time how full families' schedules can be. After 40 years of clinical experience, he now recommends telling parents to "do it as much as you can do, but at least 5 to 10 minutes a day." Most can manage that, and some will be able to do more.

Parents may ask about correcting their child's speech outside the bounds of the homework activities. Borrowing from Van Riper (1954), it may be important to tell them not to correct their child all of the time. This relieves them of the burden of having to be constantly vigilant about their child's speech, and it prevents the child from feeling they are being constantly criticized. Identifying what Van Riper called *nucleus situations* may be helpful. Perhaps a certain chair in the house or a certain activity may be labeled as the "good speech chair" or the "good speech game." It could also be a certain time of the day. The child can be told that they need to concentrate on their speech in those situations and their parents will only correct them at those times.

This also highlights the need to try to make homework practical. Sending home pictures or word lists by itself decontextualizes it and risks that it becomes just "one more thing to do." You might suggest incorporating it into their other homework routine or their bedtime preparation routine. If they are working at the connected speech level, the child could be asked to make up sentences or stories containing the target words during the ride home from school.

Generalization and Instrumental Approaches

In some of the chapters to follow, specific instrumental approaches are described. Technology is a wonderful thing, but it is not an instant answer. In the language of computer science, these approaches are *not* simply plug and play. It is not reasonable to expect that the child would be placed in front of some computerized system and instantly know how to relate to the feedback being provided on the screen. Each approach will require some initial work to orient the child to how to relate to the new feedback being provided. Some will require more orientation than others.

Related to this is the fact that there is growing evidence that the visual feedback approaches (acoustics, EPG, ultrasound) are not likely to generalize much beyond the sound in isolation level by themselves (e.g., Fletcher et al., 1991; Gibbon & Lee, 2015; McAllister Byun & Hitchcock, 2012). Therefore, in most cases it will be necessary to specifically plan for generalization when using any of these approaches.

NONSPEECH ORAL MOTOR EXERCISES

Speech is special. It is not the same as nonspeech function, and practicing nonspeech movements will not assist with speech. There is no good reason to suppose that blowing into horns, doing tongue wagging exercises, or blowing bubbles will help with speech. There are several reasons to believe this.

First, even though speech uses the same structures (i.e., nerves and muscles) as are used in nonspeech behaviors such as chewing and swallowing, the behaviors are different and are organized differently in the brain. We see this in the fact that with individuals with obvious neurological impairments, it is quite possible, for example, to have perfectly normal speech but have a swallowing disorder. Conversely, it is quite possible to have a speech disorder and have perfectly normal swallowing function. More specifically, in the adult neurological literature, it has long been known that an individual can have nonspeech oral apraxia, or apraxia of speech, or both. The fact that they can exist independently suggests they operate differently in the brain.

The second source of evidence comes from the previous discussion of motor learning principles, specifically about part versus whole practice. As a complex motor act, breaking speech down into tiny parts (that do not involve producing at least a complete speech sound) will not allow for learning of speech. We are not talking about sound shaping or phonetic placement here, which do involve producing a complete speech sound. Those are fine. However, drilling the child on tongue wagging or lip pursing or blowing whistles is not likely to generalize to speech. A complete speech sound must be included.

The third and perhaps most direct source of evidence comes from the intervention studies that have been conducted comparing the use of speech to nonspeech exercises for improving speech. Reviews of these studies by Lass and Pannbacker (2008) and Lee and Gibbon (2015) found no evidence to support their use for improving speech.

The bottom line is that practicing nonspeech behaviors that do not include complete speech sounds is not likely to be helpful for improving speech.

SUMMARY

This chapter presented some of the most recent developments in our understanding about the basic elements of treatment with a particular focus on persistent and residual /r/ errors. A major focus was on optimizing motor-based therapy. Suggestions for incorporating these suggestions into remediation efforts were provided.

In the next chapter, we revisit traditional articulation therapy and how we might fine-tune it to work more efficiently.

Motor Learning and Progress Tracking Form

Child's Name _____   Speech Target _____

Session Length _____   Session Frequency _____

Approach Used _____

	Date											
Linguistic level												
# of stimuli												
Blocked or random												
Focus (movements or output)												
KP or KR												
Feedback frequency[a]												

Total trials attempted									
% correct[a]									

Note. KP = knowledge of performance; KR = knowledge of results. Adapted from "Determining Treatment Dosage, Practice Conditions, and Feedback Methods for Speech Sound Disorders: How Do You Decide?" [Seminar presentation], by E. R. Hitchcock, M. T. Swartz, and M. Lopez, November 2019, Annual Convention of the American Speech-Language-Hearing Association, Orlando, FL.

[a]Based on last 20 trials of the session.

Notes: _____

MOTOR LEARNING AND PROGRESS TRACKING FORM EXAMPLE

Child's Name ___Noah K.___   Speech Target ___/r/ initial___

Session Length ___30 min___   Session Frequency ___2× per week___

Approach Used ___Conventional Artic.___

		Date									
	3/4/20	3/9/20	3/11/20	3/16/20	3/18/20	3/23/20	3/25/20	3/30/20			
Linguistic level	Isolation	Isolation	Syllables	Words	Words	Phrases	Phrases	Phrases			
# of stimuli	1	1	3	4	16	6	6	6			
Blocked or random	Blocked	Blocked	Blocked	Blocked	Random	Random	Random	Random			
Focus (movements or output)	Movements	Output	Output	Output	Output	Output	Output	Output			
KP or KR	KP	KR	KR	KR	KR	KR	KR	KR			
Feedback frequency[a]	80%	50%	50%	80%	25%	50%	50%	25%			

98

Total trials attempted	120	110	95	80	96	72	84	72		
% correct[a]	60%	90%	90%	80%	89%	50%	75%	90%		

Note. KP = knowledge of performance; KR = knowledge of results. Adapted from "Determining Treatment Dosage, Practice Conditicns, and Feedback Methods for Speech Sound Disorders: How Do You Decide?" [Seminar presentationl, by E. R. Hitchcock, M. T. Swartz, and M. Lopez, November 2019, Annual Convention of the American Speech-Language-Hearing Association, Orlando, FL.

[a]Based on last 20 trials of the session.

Notes: SAILS training for first 5 min of each session

CHAPTER 6

Treatment Option 1: Fine-Tuning Traditional Articulation Therapy

Our attention now turns to what most readers are interested in—specific ways to remediate /r/. The most obvious place to begin is with traditional articulation therapy. Based on both survey studies (Brumbaugh & Smit, 2013) and anecdotal reports, this appears to be what most clinicians do with clients who have residual and persistent errors. All other things being equal, it is a reasonable starting point. The main goal of this chapter, however, is to look at possible ways to use it more effectively and efficiently.

It makes sense at this point to discuss what this approach actually entails. There are at least three good reasons for doing so. First, for many of us, it has been a while since we learned about it, and it may be helpful to remind ourselves of its basic structure. A second reason is that while several alternative approaches are discussed in later chapters, those alternatives may not be accessible to some readers. For those readers, the best option may be to integrate the principles discussed in Chapter 5 with traditional therapy. Third, even for those who elect to try any of the alternatives discussed in later chapters, traditional articulation therapy is foundational to each of those alternatives. They all involve systematic variations on traditional therapy. Many, in fact, only represent tools for the initial stages of therapy that must be followed up with a systematic therapy approach such as traditional articulation therapy.

WHAT IS TRADITIONAL ARTICULATION THERAPY?

In our clinical training programs, most of us, myself included, were taught that traditional articulation therapy is attributable to Charles Van Riper.[1] Most current textbook descriptions of the approach list the following basic sequence:

1. Provide intensive ear training to deal with speech perception problems.

2. Establish the correct production of the target sound in isolation using one or more elicitation techniques.

3. Stabilize the sound in progressively longer linguistic units (syllables, words, phrases, sentences).

4. Transfer and continue maintenance (i.e., generalization) of production to conversation and everyday situations.

Many of us were also told that "almost nobody does ear training anymore." This probably explains why some current descriptions of traditional therapy do not even mention it.

Three additional dimensions of traditional therapy are often mentioned. First, some advocate that at each level (excluding spontaneous conversation), the targets should first be practiced by imitation and then spontaneously. Second, some advocate that practice at each level should first focus on each word position independently. Typically, most clinicians focus initially on consonants in initial position, then final position, and then medial position.[2] Once all three positions have been mastered, the stimuli from the different word positions are intermixed, though sources vary as to when that mixing should occur (i.e., does each word position need to be treated separately at each linguistic level, or should all the word positions be intermixed once they have been mastered at the word level?). Finally, consonants are typically practiced as singletons (i.e., without any other consonants next to them in the same syllable) before they are practiced in clusters. This last aspect is sometimes left out, and clusters are merely probed and treated separately if needed. An example of a typical treatment sequence that attempts to capture all of these dimensions (clusters excluded in this case) is shown in Table 6–1. This progression was adapted from Skelton (2004), who assumed that each word position should be treated separately at each linguistic level.

---

[1]This approach was first described in detail by Van Riper in the first (1939) edition of what became the most widely read and comprehensive textbooks in our field called *Speech Correction*. Much of the approach actually appears to also draw on the work of others including that of Lee Edward Travis (1931).

[2]There is evidence (see Kent, 1982) that for some sounds such as /s/ and /k/, production may actually be easier in final position first.

Table 6–1. Example of a Traditional Treatment Sequence for /r/

Step Number	Target
1	Perceptual training if necessary
2	Train /ɝ/ in isolation
3	Imitative trials in single syllables—initial /ɝ/
4	Imitative trials in single syllables—final /ɝ/
5	Imitative trials in disyllables—final /ɚ/
6	Imitative trials in single syllables—initial /r/
7	Imitative trials in single syllables—final /r/
8	Imitative trials in single words—initial /ɝ/
9	Imitative trials in single words—final /ɝ/
10	Imitative trials in single words—final /ɚ/
11	Imitative trials in single words—initial /r/
12	Imitative trials in single words—final /r/
13	Spontaneous trials in single words—initial /ɝ/
14	Spontaneous trials in single words—final /ɝ/
15	Spontaneous trials in single words—final /ɚ/
16	Spontaneous trials in single words—initial /r/
17	Spontaneous trials in single words—final /r/
18	Imitative trials in two- to four-word phrases—initial /ɝ/
19	Imitative trials in two- to four-word phrases—final /ɝ/
20	Imitative trials in two- to four-word phrases—final /ɚ/
21	Imitative trials in two- to four-word phrases—initial /r/
22	Imitative trials in two- to four-word phrases—final /r/
23	Spontaneous trials in two- to four-word phrases—initial /ɝ/
24	Spontaneous trials in two- to four-word phrases—final /ɝ/
25	Spontaneous trials in two- to four-word phrases—final /ɚ/
26	Spontaneous trials in two- to four-word phrases—initial /r/
27	Spontaneous trials in two- to four-word phrases—final /r/
28	Imitative trials in single sentences—initial /ɝ/

continues

Table 6–1. *continued*

Step Number	Target
29	Imitative trials in single sentences—final /ɝ/
30	Imitative trials in single sentences—final /ɚ/
31	Imitative trials in single sentences—initial /r/
32	Imitative trials in single sentences—final /r/
33	Spontaneous trials in single sentences—initial /ɝ/
34	Spontaneous trials in single sentences—final /ɝ/
35	Spontaneous trials in single sentences—final /ɚ/
36	Spontaneous trials in single sentences—initial /r/
37	Spontaneous trials in single sentences—final /r/
38	Spontaneous conversation—all forms of /r/

Note. Adapted from Table 2 in "Concurrent Task Sequencing in Single-Phoneme Phonologic Treatment and Generalization," by S. L. Skelton, 2004, *Journal of Communication Disorders*, *37*, p. 136 (https://doi.org/10.1016/j.jcomdis.2003.08.002).

How does this compare to what Van Riper proposed? In the 1954 (third) edition of his book, Van Riper provided an outline that included seven steps[3]:

1. The speech defective must be convinced that he has errors that he must eradicate.

2. The causes of the disorder, if still existent, must be eliminated. If those causes are no longer present, their influence must be counteracted.

3. Through intensive ear training, the old word configurations are broken down so that correct sound may be isolated, recognized, identified, and discriminated.

4. Through various methods, the speech defective must be taught to produce the correct sound in isolation and at will.

5. The new and correct sound must be strengthened.

---

[3]With the exception of some changes in terminology and more detail about linguistic levels, the description of the approach remained largely unchanged through the last (ninth) edition of the book (Van Riper & Erickson, 1996), which appeared shortly after Van Riper's death in 1994.

6. The new sound must be incorporated within familiar words, and the transition to normal speech must be accomplished.

7. The use of the correct sound must be made habitual, and the error must be eliminated. (p. 205)

If one considers the publication date, Van Riper might be excused, if not forgiven, for his somewhat outdated (and in some cases clearly derogatory) terminology. That aside, notice that ear training is not even the first step. As well, in the last edition of his book (Van Riper & Erickson, 1996), Steps 1 and 2 are not included in the initial description but are discussed separately.

Looking at his Step 1, Van Riper (1954) noted that it is necessary to ensure that the child is motivated to change what they are doing. Motivation was discussed in Chapter 5 under prepractice goals, but that discussion assumed a child who has already agreed to participate in therapy. Recall, however, the discussion of evidence-based practice (EBP) in Chapter 1, where as children get older (although parents make the ultimate decision), they should be asked to give their assent to treatment. For the child who is teased about their speech errors, little motivation may be needed, though they may need to balance that against any teasing that comes with attending therapy. In cases where there are no negative peer inputs, however, the older child who does not see the need to change is less likely to cooperate in therapy, and change is less likely to happen. Van Riper (1954) admits how difficult it can be to try to convince a child (who does not already recognize it) that they have speech errors that need correcting. He does point out that in order to do so, it will be necessary to point out their specific errors. He says that "(a) vague, generalized feeling that something is wrong with speech will not provide sufficient motivation" (p. 206). For older children, some of the self-assessment and self-monitoring activities discussed in Chapter 5 might be useful at the very beginning of therapy to help increase their motivation to change.

The second step prior to beginning ear training, according to Van Riper, is the elimination of causal factors, something most current clinicians would take almost as a given. This issue was discussed in Chapter 4 under factors to consider and in Chapter 5 under prepractice goals. Clearly, significant structural and motor differences may require medical referral. Minor structural and motor issues are unlikely to be impacting the production of single sound errors, but hearing and visual acuity impairments must be addressed.

That brings us to Step 3, ear training. Although this reflected the thinking at the time that all children with speech sound disorders have a perceptual problem, its use remained part of Van Riper's description of the approach even in the 1996 edition of his book. We now know that perceptual intervention may not be necessary in all cases. However, as discussed in Chapters 4 and 5, where perceptual testing indicates a problem, some sort of perceptual therapy would appear to be warranted.

Step 4 is really where most of us currently begin. We look to teach the production of the sound by itself. For the child who is stimulable for their error, this step may not involve much work, but for those who are not, the elicitation of a fully correct /r/ may be a challenge. Thankfully, there are many techniques available to assist with this. These are discussed relative to /r/ later in this chapter.

It is likely that Step 5, the strengthening of the new and correct sound, is not discussed much these days. According to Van Riper (1954), it involves two parts. The first is the use of the sound by itself in a variety of ways such as prolongation, repetition, exaggeration, and simultaneous talking and writing. Van Riper describes the last procedure as the most important. The child is asked to handwrite the letter (note that he only mentions and shows script not printed forms) at the exact time that they produce the sound. He claims that it will "not only provide an excellent vehicle for practice of the new sound, but also give a means of reinforcing the motor aspect of performance" (p. 250). Van Riper also suggests that the student can do this on their own as a homework activity.

The second part of strengthening (Step 5) mentioned by Van Riper is practice in nonsense material. Although this step is occasionally discussed as a way to overcome bad habits that emerge at the word level, it is often mentioned only as an optional intermediate step between the isolation and word levels. Brumbaugh and Smit (2013) found that only 34% of clinicians reported using this step.[4] Van Riper notes that practice in nonsense syllables allows for practice of the target sound in a wide variety of other sound contexts (e.g., with a variety of vowels). Later our field would come to refer to this as coarticulation, which was discussed in Chapter 2. One benefit noted by Van Riper for the use of nonsense material is that it will always be new to the child. That means the child will only be practicing the correct version of the sound. Given the amount of time these children spend practicing their errors outside of therapy, this can only be a good thing. Van Riper suggested that practice here start with the sound in initial position (e.g., /ro/, /rʌ/, /rɑ/), then final position (e.g., /ir/, /ɛr/, /ur/), and last medial position (e.g., /ɑrɑ/). He notes that reduplicated syllables (e.g., /roro/ or /irir/) could also be included.

Step 6 as delineated by Van Riper (1954) involves using real words and transitioning to real speech. Personal experience and reports from other clinicians suggest that this can be a difficult step with children who

---

[4]Brumbaugh and Smit (2013) were surveying clinicians serving preschoolers. The lesser use of nonsense materials with young children is not surprising given that young children often have difficulty relating to nonsense material. Their use with older children is not clear.

have strongly ingrained errors. However, Van Riper noted that "(i)f the preliminary work has been done carefully, there will be little difficulty" (p. 253). That said, he offered several suggestions for managing the transition. These include activities such as *reconfiguration*, which involves gradual integration of the new sound into its proper place in words. It could start with practicing a substitution of another already correct sound for the target sound. For example, they could substitute /b/ for /r/ while reading words or short sentences. They could say, "Bay is going fishing" instead of "Ray is going fishing" or "I see a bed circle" instead of "I see a red circle." After lots of practice with various stimuli, another transition step would be to substitute the new target sound for a different sound such as saying /r/ whenever /s/ was intended as in "Rammy is ritting at the table" instead of "Sammy is sitting at the table." A third transition step might be to omit all of the intended /r/ sounds. In this case, they would say "_yan has a _ed ca_" instead of "Ryan has a red car." Finally, they would be asked to insert the correct sound. It is noteworthy that each of these suggestions effectively requires segmentation of the words, which was one of the phonological awareness tasks described previously. As such, Van Riper was, perhaps unknowingly, strengthening the underlying representation for the speech sound and helping to mitigate potential reading problems. One additional transition suggestion mentioned by Van Riper might serve the same end. It is to repeat the *simultaneous talking and writing* procedure mentioned earlier but using real words and sentences this time.

Finally, for Step 7, Van Riper (1954) notes that the child "must follow a systematic program of effecting the transition into casual speech" (p. 256). This is what is now called programming for generalization. Much of what was discussed about generalization in Chapter 5 was drawn from the work of Van Riper. For this step, Van Riper specifically mentions speech assignments (i.e., homework) for the child to carry out where they deliberately focus on their speech sound production and report back at the next session. Such activities might include the child asking others (a parent, another familiar adult, a trusted peer, or older sibling) to give them feedback about their speech during a few minutes of conversation. It could also include asking them to try to deliberately insert specific words they have been practicing in therapy into their conversations with others.

CURRENT PRACTICE VERSUS VAN RIPER'S APPROACH

In addition to listing a different set of steps (see the start of this chapter), current descriptions of traditional articulation therapy differ from the approach advocated by Van Riper in at least three other respects. First, as already discussed, most clinicians appear to have abandoned the practice of ear training for every child, and they tend to focus solely on production. Second, for those who follow a sequence similar to that shown in Table 6–1, imitation is used to begin each linguistic level; Van Riper only mentioned imitation at the isolation and syllable level. Finally, some suggest treating each word position separately at each linguistic level; Van Riper describes a process in which, starting at the word level, one word position is used initially. Once mastered at that level, a second word position is introduced and added to the practice material from the first word position. Then a third word position is introduced and added to the practice material. Finally, if appropriate, clusters are added. Over time, the practice material expands to include multiple contexts. Thus, generalization is being planned for at this early stage. At all subsequent levels (phrases, sentences, conversation), all word positions and clusters are intermixed in therapy. This approach is consistent with the recommendation on practice variability from Chapter 5.

If traditional articulation therapy differs from what clinicians currently do, how does one reconcile that? Should we simply go back to what Van Riper suggested? Or should we follow the lead of current clinicians who may have intuitively figured out a better way? Rather than do either, it makes sense to look at the available evidence. What has empirical research shown us about what does and does not work in traditional articulation therapy?

EVIDENCE IN SUPPORT OF TRADITIONAL THERAPY

It is worth starting out with a general statement. No matter how it is being administered, traditional therapy seems to work. It may not be 100% successful for all children, but in general it works. Countless clinicians will attest to its value, and a considerable body of empirical evidence supports its use (see Preston & Leece, 2021, for a review). Some specific examples of studies conducted over the past five decades include Carrier (1970), Evans and Potter (1974), Gunther and Hautvast (2010), Helmick (1976), Hesketh, Adams, Nightingale, and Hall (2000), Rvachew and Brosseau-Lepre (2015), and Sommers and colleagues (1967).

As for the specific components of this approach, not all have been examined, and there is spotty evidence for those components that have. However, there is a good deal to be learned from reviewing what evidence is available. Note that some of the studies described later in this chapter did not specifically involve traditional articulation therapy but were included because they happened to include a component that is also used in traditional therapy.

The question of whether ear training (perceptual therapy) is necessary was addressed in Chapter 4. To summarize, it is clearly not required for all children, but in cases where perceptual deficits occur, it makes sense to include it.

The requirement to follow a hierarchy of therapy across isolation, syllables, words, sentences, and conversation is described by Van Riper and Erickson (1996) as "(t)he hallmark of traditional articulation therapy" (p. 237). That said, are all the steps necessary? Practicing clinicians do not appear to be convinced that they are. In their survey, Brumbaugh and Smit (2013) reported that 82% of clinicians used traditional articulation therapy sometimes, often, or always (i.e., at least 40% of the time) to treat speech sound disorders. However, depending on the specific step, those same clinicians reported using them anywhere from 34% of the time for nonsense syllables to 86% of the time for words in treatment.

Evidence for the need for specific steps in the hierarchy is limited, and findings are somewhat mixed. Looking at generalization across levels, McReynolds (1972) reported findings from four children ages 6;1 to 8;3 who were producing errors on /s/. Training in isolation did not transfer to the word level, but such transfer did start once practice in the initial position of nonsense syllables was introduced. Transfer did not generalize to other word positions until continuous reinforcement was replaced with feedback on every third attempt (this effectively meant the children had to self-monitor their other attempts). The introduction of training in the final position of nonsense syllables did not result in any more generalization, which did not occur until training in the medial position of nonsense syllables began. These results suggest that training in isolation and nonsense syllables is required for success at the word level. On the other hand, a study by Irwin and colleagues (1976) involving 369 children ages 6 to 15 years (mostly for /s/ errors; other targets were not specified) found that a paired-stimuli approach involving training only at the word level was successful for 338 (92%) of the children. Thus, training below the word level may not always be needed.

There is some evidence suggesting that if the steps are all needed, it may not be necessary to follow them in any particular order. Findings from several studies of *concurrent treatment* by Skelton and colleagues (see further discussion in Chapter 7) suggest that completely randomizing the order of training can yield significant improvement (e.g., Skelton, 2004). However, only one (as yet unpublished) study has compared the randomized order to the traditional order, so it is not clear if outcomes with a randomized order are any more efficacious than the standard order.

Van Riper advocated for imitation to precede spontaneous productions, at least during the earliest stage of therapy. However, there is limited evidence to support such a general requirement. In a treatment study with two preschool children using a minimal pairs approach targeting one fricative each, Saben and Ingham (1991) reported little to no progress until imitation trials were introduced. This suggests the need for such imitation training. On the other hand, Skelton (2004) included a mix of imitative and spontaneous trials presented randomly and reported success suggesting that imitation need not occur before requiring spontaneous productions. Both studies included small samples, which may indicate that the need for imitation as an initial step may vary across individuals.

As mentioned earlier, where it is used, Van Riper's descriptions do not appear to mention imitation above the syllable level. Van Riper appeared to be a strong advocate for practicing speech in natural communicative contexts, and it would be hard to argue that imitation at the word level and above is a natural way to communicate. No specific evidence for its use or nonuse above the syllable level appears to be available.

The question of needing to treat by individual word positions has also received some limited attention. Ruscello (1975) studied six children ages 6;7 to 9;1 with /s/ misarticulations. Three children (Group I) received therapy focused on initial position only, while the focus of treatment for the other three (Group II) included all three word positions from the very beginning. Overall performance was greater for Group II who also showed consistently higher performance across all three word positions. A narrow focus on one word position may not be optimal. Another study by Weaver-Spurlock and Brasseur (1988) used a multiple baseline across participants' research design to treat three children ages 5;0 to 5;7 with /s/ errors using practice at all three word positions simultaneously. Generalization to untreated words (and to a lesser extent to conversation) occurred for all three children. Together these findings suggest that a narrow focus on a single word position may not be optimal and that a focus on multiple word positions simultaneously may be of greater value. This is consistent with the notion of a possible advantage for random practice discussed under principles of motor learning in Chapter 5.

From the very beginning of the therapy process, Van Riper empha-sized the need for the child to be aware of their errors and to be able to identify those errors when they occur. This is what is currently termed *self-monitoring*. A few studies have examined this aspect of therapy. A 1986 study by Koegel, Koegel, and Ingham involved 13 children ages 6;6 to 10;9 with errors on either /s, z/ or /r/. Four of the children had received previous treatment. Using a multiple baseline across participants design, self-monitoring was introduced at different points in the therapy process for each child (i.e., some started it as they reached the sentence level, some did not start it until they reached the conversation level). The children were trained to listen for and record the accuracy of their productions in conversational interactions in the treatment sessions. No self-monitoring was required outside of treatment. Generalization to speech outside of therapy was measured by outside observers (not the treating clinician). All of the children were 0% correct in conversation outside of therapy until the self-monitoring training was introduced in therapy. Accuracy in outside conversation then quickly increased to over 90% for 9/13 children. This suggested that, regardless of the point in therapy where it is introduced, training self-monitoring within the treatment sessions can stimulate generalization outside of therapy in many cases. Another study by Gray and Shelton (1992) yielded conflicting findings. That study involved eight children ages 7;7 to 12;4 being treated for /s/ or /r/ errors. All had received some previous treatment and had already achieved at least 60% correct for the target sound in conversation in the clinic setting. Five of the eight were less than 40% correct in conversation outside of the clinic setting, while the other three were above 80%. Self-monitoring was taught, and the children were required to tally each correct instance of their target sound on a wrist counter during three time periods outside therapy. Findings indicated that the addition of self-monitoring did not assist with generalization to conversation outside of therapy. Differences in the way these two studies were conducted may have accounted for the conflicting results. None of the children in the study by Koegel and colleagues were yet generalizing to conversational speech (within therapy), whereas all of the children in the Gray and Shelton study were doing so. It is conceivable that introducing self-monitoring for children who are not yet generalizing to conversation may be of some assistance with generalization to outside settings.

The final aspect of traditional therapy that has received some empirical examination is the use of homework assignments. This is considered a major element in generalization beyond the therapy room in Van Riper's approach as well as in some other treatment approaches. Intuitively, it makes sense that it would be very helpful, but here again, limited study of it appears to have been conducted. A German study by Gunther and Hautvast (2010) compared three groups of children ages 4 to 6 years. A control group of 26 children on a waiting list received no intervention. The two treatment groups received traditional articulation therapy for /s/ and/or /ʃ/ consisting of eight 45-min sessions over 4 weeks. Homework was assigned to both treatment groups, and all children were required to report on how much of the homework activities they had done. No other element was added for one group ($n = 32$), while the third group ($n = 33$) was provided with individual rewards (a token system where tokens could be exchanged for prizes) for recording their homework. The control group was relatively unchanged over the treatment period, but both treatment groups improved significantly, again supporting the efficacy of traditional therapy. On a 33-item probe, the group without rewards improved from a mean of 32.2 errors to a mean of 7.8 errors. The group with rewards improved from 32.3 errors to 3.0 errors, which was a statistically larger improvement suggesting that the addition of the reward system aided in generalization. Findings from this one study only demonstrate that where homework is used, reward systems can make it more effective. No clear evidence appears to be available on the benefits of homework itself.

Box 6–1: Summary of Evidence for Traditional Articulation Therapy

It works!

Perceptual training is only needed for documented perceptual deficits.

Strict adherence to the order of the treatment hierarchy may not be necessary.

Treatment below the word level may not always be needed.

Imitation may only be needed for some children.

Where needed, it may only be needed below the word level.

A focus on a single word position may not be needed (including a mixed set of word positions may be more efficient).

Training self-monitoring may be of value only for children who are not yet generalizing to the conversation level.

Homework may be helpful.

Where used, adding a reward system may make homework more effective.

Assuming an EBP perspective, it makes sense to apply that evidence to our understanding of how traditional articulation therapy should be conducted. Combining that with the principles of motor learning discussed in Chapter 5 would yield what should be a more efficient treatment sequence for /r/, which is now shown in Table 6–2.

Note that the sequence in Table 6–2 represents a significant reduction in steps from the 38 steps in Table 6–1. Such a reduction alone might render therapy less cumbersome.

Such a treatment sequence could be instituted immediately following a baseline probe that would be recorded to serve as the basis for monitoring progress and checking for generalization. This might involve conducting a stimulability probe as in shown in Appendix 4–1 and measuring accuracy in conversation using the form in Appendix 4–3. Administering a single-word probe such as is shown in Table 4–1 might also be worth considering. The particular words in that probe would then need to be excluded from therapy sessions.

Table 6–2. Traditional Articulation Therapy Treatment Sequence Adjusted to Account for Available Evidence and Principles of Motor Learning

Step Number	Target
1	Perceptual training if necessary
2	Train /ɝ/ in isolation—provide knowledge of performance feedback
3	Imitative trials in single syllables—initial /ɝ/
4	Imitative trials in single syllables—initial /ɝ/ + final /ɝ/ – reduce feedback to every other trial
5	Imitative trials in single syllables—initial /ɝ/ + final /ɝ/ + disyllables – final /ɚ/
6	Imitative trials in single syllables—initial /ɝ/ + final /ɝ/ + initial /r/ + disyllables – final /ɚ/
7	Imitative trials in single syllables—initial /ɝ/ + final /ɝ/ + initial /r/ + final /r/ + disyllables – final /ɚ/
8	Spontaneous trials in single words—initial /ɝ/ – switch to knowledge of results feedback
9	Spontaneous trials in single words—initial /ɝ/ + final /ɝ/
10	Spontaneous trials in single words—initial /ɝ/ + final /ɝ/ + final /ɚ/ – feedback every fifth trial
11	Spontaneous trials in single words—initial /ɝ/ + final /ɝ/ + final /ɚ/ + initial /r/
12	Spontaneous trials in single words—initial /ɝ/ + final /ɝ/ + final /ɚ/ + initial /r/ + final /r/
13	Train self-monitoring
14	Introduce homework
15	Spontaneous trials in two- to four-word phrases—all forms of /r/
16	Spontaneous trials in clinician-generated single sentences—all forms of /r/
17	Spontaneous trials in self-generated single sentences—all forms of /r/
18	Spontaneous conversation—all forms of /r/

Note. Adapted from Table 2 in "Concurrent Task Sequencing in Single-Phoneme Phonologic Treatment and Generalization," by S. L. Skelton, 2004, *Journal of Communication Disorders,* *37,* p. 136 (https://doi.org/10.1016/j.jcomdis.2003.08.002) and Table 6–1 herein.

ELICITING A GOOD /r/

Sequence and steps aside, no approach to remediating /r/ (or any speech sound for that matter) will be successful if the child is unable to produce the target sound consistently correctly. For the child who is not stimulable for /r/, getting them to produce a good /r/ remains a significant challenge for clinicians. One of the best available sources is the widely used book, *Eliciting Sounds* by Wayne Secord and colleagues (2007). It includes a wide range of techniques specific to /r/. Another useful resource is Bleile's (2018) book, *The Late Eight*, which also includes an array of procedures for eliciting /r/. Both are strongly recommended.

Facilitating Contexts for /r/

Before discussing the teaching of the target sound in isolation, starting at a higher level such as the word level might be considered. It has been suggested over the years that if the right context can be found, the lower levels can be avoided. An early sense of this is found in the *coarticulation approach* of Eugene McDonald (1964). The concept is discussed in detail by Kent (1982), who defined *facilitating contexts* as "certain phonetic environments or linguistic conditions [that] are more likely than others to be associated with correct sound production" (p. 66). As a general rule, for example, Kent noted that "(i)t seems advisable to work with the error sound in stressed syllables, first" (p. 67), as the target is easier to hear both in models from the clinician and by the child in their own speech. More specific to /r/, he commented that it may be more likely to be correct in words containing initial clusters rather than initial singletons. In particular, /r/ produced in initial /dr/, /gr/, /tr/, and /kr/ contexts (in that rank order) may be more likely to elicit correct productions. Kent offers several possible explanations for this. The first is that by starting with stop consonants, these contexts provide more definitive tactile feedback than /r/ by itself. Likewise, the tongue-tip elevation for the alveolars (/dr, tr/) may lead naturally to a retroflex /r/ production, while the tongue-dorsum elevation for the velars (/gr, kr/) may lead more naturally to a bunched /r/ production. Given what we know about how different speakers appear to have a preference for one or the other of these tongue shapes, you should not be surprised to hear that, in my experience, I have noted that some children respond better to the alveolar context, while others respond better to the velar context. Kent also notes that the voiced contexts (/dr, gr/) may be preferable because the additional loudness of voiced consonants makes them easier to hear than the voiceless contexts (/tr, kr/). In addition to the cluster context, Kent (1982) also noted that vowel context should also be considered. Back vowels (e.g., /u, o/) include lip rounding that may inadvertently stimulate the common error [w], likely because /w/ also includes lip approximation. To put it another way, the presence of back vowels may tend to bring out the old error. Front vowels would therefore be preferable. Taken together, this would suggest that words like *dream, dress, dry, green,* and *gray* might be more likely to elicit a correct /r/.

A question that arises relative to facilitating context relates to next steps. Assuming a correct production can be elicited with such a context, how does one generalize the correct production to other contexts? This would require the slow introduction of other contexts. For example, Kent (1982) offers an extended list of the next most facilitating contexts, which would be (in order): /ri/, /br/, /pr/, /ru/, /rɑ/, and /fr/. These could each be introduced one at a time. Central vowel and back vowel contexts could also slowly be introduced.

The *Systematic Articulation Training Program Accessing Computers* (SATPAC) approach (discussed in Chapter 7) attempts to take advantage of facilitating contexts within a nonsense material framework to help get around old habits and try to establish new ones. This is consistent with the previously described notion of strengthening the production (Van Riper's Step 5) by using nonsense syllables. For example, a common context used in SATPAC for /r/ is the nonsense syllable "eergah" (/irgæ/). The combination of an initial front vowel combined with a voiced velar stop is intended to simulate the motion of producing a bunched /r/ between two different vowels (a more dynamic gesture than producing /r/ in isolation).

While this approach has some appeal and is used, direct comparisons of starting with facilitating contexts at the word level versus starting at the isolation level do not appear to have been conducted. Lacking such evidence, most clinicians appear to prefer starting at the isolated sound level. There are a number of procedures available for doing so with /r/.

Modeling a Good /r/

Advocates of starting with sounds in isolation almost always note that this should be first attempted using *imitation*. This is sometimes referred to as *auditory stimulation* as it involves providing an auditory model. Although less likely for those with long-established habits, for some clients, providing them with a good model and asking them to repeat may be enough. The idea is to then give them feedback on their production and see if they can figure out what to do with their vocal tract on their own. Most sources (see also Table 6–2) start with a stressed vocalic /ɝ/.

The use of imitation presumes that a good model is being provided. Box 6–2 presents some general suggestions for doing this. These are based on several sources including Miccio (2002) and personal conversations with several clinician-researchers. A comment about the last point in Box 6–2 is warranted. Recall from Chapter 1 the discussion of the challenges of /r/

and demographic dynamics. Acoustically, the models we provide to our clients differ from what they might produce because of adult–child and male–female differences in vocal tract size and configuration. These differences may make it more difficult for our clients to effectively make use of those models. As such, it might be worth considering making recordings of speech models from same-age and same-gender peers of your client to minimize the potential impact of such differences. How important this might be is unknown at this time.

Box 6–2: Suggestions for Modeling a Good /ɝ/

Initially provide a model before each attempt.

Do not exaggerate lip rounding.

Use normal voice volume.

Prolong for no more than 1 to 1.5 s (prevents a tendency to focus only on length and miss relevant acoustic cues).

See also Appendix 4–1 for modeling instructions.

Consider using recorded models from same-age and same-gender peers.

Specific Elicitation Procedures

Beyond imitation, a common approach to elicitation is the use of *phonetic placement* procedures. These involve describing to our client how to produce the speech sound target. This might be accomplished with words, pictures, and/or hand gestures to illustrate to the child what the articulators are doing when a correct version of the target sound is produced. In the case of /r/, given the discussion in Chapter 2, the basic information that is being conveyed likely needs to change. At the very least, we should be prepared to include both retroflex and bunched tongue shapes. In most cases, one of these would be trialed and if it were unsuccessful, we would switch to the other.

Until recently, most discussions of eliciting /r/ have not mentioned the pharyngeal constriction. Preston and Leece (2019) suggested instructions such as "pretend you are holding a marble in between your tongue and the back of the throat" or "pull the back of your tongue way into the back of your throat." Talking about tongue bracing or at least the tactile feedback of the tongue contacting the upper back teeth might be of some value where a bunched /r/ tongue shape is being targeted. Conversely, with a retroflex tongue shape target, it may be helpful to ask the child to think about the sides of the tongue touching the lower back teeth while the tongue tip is raised.

Productions of a bunched /r/ might be elicited by asking the child to first place their tongue tip behind their lower front teeth. Then ask them to raise the body of the tongue up toward the roof of the mouth (somewhat similar to producing /k/). Then we would have them imitate /ɝ/.

Productions of a retroflex /r/ could be elicited by asking them to put their tongue tip up behind their front teeth. Then they would be asked to curl their tongue backward while imitating /ɝ/.

Visual images are sometimes helpful in phonetic placement instruction. These could include the diagrams from Chapter 2. The book by Secord and colleagues (2007) includes similar diagrams. More recently, digital programs have been developed such as one called *Sounds of Speech*. It was developed by the University of Iowa Research Foundation (2016) originally as a website (https://soundsofspeech.uiowa.edu/home), but it is now available as a tablet and phone-based app at the App Store and Google Play. It includes simple animations to demonstrate how speech sounds are typically produced. It should be noted that relative to /r/, it only presents an animation for a bunched /r/. Another example called Pronunciation Coach is available from Rose Medical (http://rose-medical .com/pronunciation-coach.html). One advantage of this program is that in addition to showing sounds in isolation, words can be entered and the software then produces an animation of the entire word. In addition, it allows you to adjust the rate of speech from fairly slow to fairly fast to allow for closer examination of the movements involved. It is a Windows-based program only, however, and it is limited by only using a bunched /r/.

Phonetic placement procedures may also include some physical manipulation of the articulators. For example, a tongue depressor may be used to lift up the tongue tip for a retroflex /r/ or to push the tongue tip down for a bunched /r/.

It is noteworthy that in their treatment study using visual acoustic feedback, Shuster, Ruscello, and Smith (1992) noted that general instructions about phonetic placement for /r/ may not be sufficient for some clients because of the across-speaker and across-context variability in the way normal /r/ is produced. They suggested that more specific instruction such as sound shaping may be more useful.

That then leads us to a discussion of *sound shaping*, which is perhaps the most widely used approach. It is also referred to as *sound approximation*. These procedures may involve starting with a nonspeech sound such as the growl of an angry tiger. More often the /r/ target may also be shaped from any number of speech sounds that the child already produces correctly. For example, Shriberg (1975) presented a detailed procedure for shaping /r/ from /l/. Bleile (2018) offers steps for shaping /r/ from /ð/ or from /ɑ/. Stephen Sacks has developed his own approach to eliciting /r/

using multisyllabic nonwords. Whatever the starting point, it is then modified in a series of small steps or gradual movements so that it becomes /r/. Specific instructions for each of these procedures are provided in Appendix 6–1.

Cues for Fine-Tuning Production

In addition to eliciting those initial correct productions, additional cues may be helpful for continued correct production. Several different kinds of cues have been documented.

Metaphors

Although not a specific elicitation technique, Bleile (2018) and others have suggested that correct production may be assisted by using verbal metaphors while conducting elicitation activities. These metaphors are useful ways to describe the sound being produced and would be introduced early to evoke mental images about what is happening in the mouth. They could also be used later in therapy as reminders whenever errors occur. As with so many other aspects of traditional therapy, there do not appear to have been any empirical studies of the use of these.

Specific to /r/, Bleile (2018) suggests metaphors that evoke images of the /r/ quality of the sound such as a "growling sound" or a "pirate sound"). He also suggests other metaphors that evoke images about tongue placement ("tongue tip flat sound" for a bunched /r/; "tongue tip up sound" for a retroflex /r/).

Touch Cues

Another supplement to elicitation documented by Bleile (2018) is the use of touch cues. These represent signals that the child is taught to do in which their own hand is placed in somewhat static positions at various points around the face to reinforce the placement or movement of the tongue inside the mouth. As with metaphors, these would be used during elicitation and could be revived later in therapy as reminders about correct production. Again, no empirical studies could be identified to support or refute the use of these.

For /r/, Bleile (2018) suggests having the child place their hand on one side of the mouth. If the target is a bunched /r/, the child's palm is face down and the fingertips are curled under as a signal to keep the tongue tip down. If the target is a retroflex /r/, the child's palm is face up, and the fingertips are curled facing up. This serves as a reminder to keep the tongue tip up.

Gestural Cues

A number of sources over the years have suggested the addition of gestures or hand movements to supplement other therapy activities. The idea is to provide visual and/or kinesthetic cues for correct production of the targets. Some suggested examples include tracing a finger along the arm to imitate the continuous airflow in the production of a fricative such as /s/ or a fist being quickly opened up to demonstrate the release of pressure for a stop consonant such as /p/. Relative to /r/, Ristuccia (2002) suggested the addition of a hand gesture in which the fingers are pulled back from the horizontal (similar to squeezing a ball from the top) to simulate a bunched /r/.

Although empirical study of the efficacy of using gestures for remediating speech errors has been very limited, one study appears relevant here. It was a 2017 single-subject study by Rusiewicz and Rivera involving a 21-year-old woman with persistent childhood apraxia of speech. The focus was on the production of postvocalic /r/. The patient had a long history of therapy from 4 to 18 years of age but presented with a consistently derhotacized (distorted) /r/. Over three baseline sessions with no treatment, her accuracy for correct /r/ remained at 0%. Then therapy was introduced involving phonetic placement instruction, CV stimuli written out on cards, combined with a hand gesture simulating a bunched /r/. The gesture used appears to have been almost identical to the one from Ristuccia (2002) described earlier. The patient was told that the fingertips represented the tip of the tongue and the hand movement represented the overall movement of the tongue; she was encouraged to produce the hand gesture along with her production attempts. After five 30-min treatment sessions, accuracy increased from 0% to over 70%. At that point, treatment was paused and accuracy was the monitored over four sessions. Her performance decreased to approximately 30%. Therapy was then reintroduced, and accuracy improved to 100% after three additional sessions and remained at that level for three follow-up sessions. These findings strongly suggested that the combination of the gesture and other therapy activities was responsible for the changes.

JAW STABILIZATION

Some advocates of nonspeech oral motor exercises (e.g., Borshart, 2016) have proposed using activities and/or devices that enhance the stability of the tongue or jaw. Nonspeech oral motor exercises were discussed in general in Chapter 5 and are not necessarily being advocated here. However, some discussion of jaw stabilization may be relevant to /r/.

Producing speech sounds requires consistently placing the various parts of the vocal tract into specific positions. It has been suggested that some children may have difficulty doing so. For example, Dworkin (1978) reported on four boys ages 6;7 to 8;0 who produced distorted alveolar consonants that were "often accompanied by hypermandibular activity (HMA); they intermittently demonstrated exaggerated mandibular excursions that appeared to interfere particularly with the differential valving action of the tongue" (p. 169). In other words, they were unable to consistently place and maintain the jaw in the required position for some speech sounds, and this appeared to interfere with tongue placement.

Assuming some children with speech sound disorders have this problem, what might explain such difficulties? At least two accounts are possible. One possibility is that problems with jaw positioning represent an underlying disorder or delay in the development of fine motor control of the jaw. This may be the case, but specific published evidence for such deficits or delays is lacking for children with speech sound disorders in general or for those with /r/ errors in particular. An alternative explanation (also without specific published evidence to support it) is that some children have a temporary sensory awareness issue. The logic goes like this. Think back to your first phonetics class. For most readers, this was probably the first time they were asked to consider what was happening inside their own mouth during speech. Even as a competent, typically speaking adult, it probably took some time to develop a solid awareness of what was happening. It might also be a similar situation for children with speech sound disorders. When they first enter therapy, it is not uncommon to observe them struggling or groping, at least initially, when asked to perform specific speech activities. They are being asked to sort out feedback from the articulators that previously were not given much conscious attention. For most, as therapy progresses, they become more skilled at sorting out this feedback and better at performing the movements required of them. It is possible that some children have more difficulty than others with sorting out this feedback. Given the challenges described for the production of /r/ (e.g., three constrictions, limited tactile feedback), it would not be a surprise that this difficulty may be especially acute for this sound.

Whatever the explanation, the use of jaw stabilization activities or devices for remediating /r/ offers another potential benefit. By temporarily stabilizing the jaw (fixing it in one position), feedback from jaw motion is removed, and the child may be better able to focus their attention on the critical feedback needed from the tongue and/or pharynx to allow them to make the two oral constrictions (palatal and pharyngeal) for /r/. This is similar to the justification often given for using a bite block or bite stick with adults who have acquired neurological impairments. Duffy (2005) states that "a bite block could be used to 'force' increased lip and tongue movement during therapy activities by taking jaw movements out of the speech loop" (p. 477). For children with speech sound disorders, where typically no neurological deficit can be documented, such devices may be helping them to disentangle all of the sensory information involved in producing this most complex sound.

Regardless of the explanation, the suggestion to use a bite-stick to assist with children is not a new idea. Shriberg (1980) suggested the use of 4- to 6-in.-long dowel of wood perhaps three-eighths inch in diameter (a standard pencil or pen would also work) specifically for remediating /r/. He mentions that the clinician could demonstrate on themselves before introducing it. Although Shriberg (1980) did not present any empirical data to support the use of such devices, a limited amount of data are available that appear to support their use. A case study by Flipsen and Sacks (2015) using the SATPAC approach (discussed in Chapter 7) included the use of three tongue depressors taped together and held flat between the teeth at the side of the mouth. The child was able to establish a consistent /r/, and their errors were successfully remediated with the rest of the program. The second source of evidence comes from the previously cited paper by Dworkin (1978), which was a treatment study. Productions of all alveolar consonants (/t, d, n, l, s, z/) for the four children were described as distorted, and 3 months of prior therapy had not resulted in any improvement. Therapy using a one-half-inch round plastic bite-block (with attached handle) was introduced; holding it between the teeth provided a stabilized jaw and allowed for practice of independent movements of the tongue tip. All four children successfully corrected all of their errors in 40 to 48 treatment sessions (60 min each). Another example of the use of jaw stabilization is Speech Buddies®, which are intraoral devices that require the client to hold them between their teeth. The part that projects into the mouth assists with tongue placement and/or movement, but the act of holding the device in their teeth provides jaw stabilization. As discussed in Chapter 8, there is some evidence suggesting these devices can help with speech sound remediation. Together these findings suggest that jaw stabilization may be of some assistance with some children. Its use with remediating /r/ would appear to be at least worth considering. A simple bite-block can be made by taping three tongue blades together as shown in Figure 6–1.

ALTERNATIVE FEEDBACK

The procedures discussed earlier assume conventional verbal feedback is being provided. In other words, the speech-language pathologist (SLP) provides instructions, the client tries to carry them out, and the SLP tells them specifically what they did or did not do correctly (i.e., provides knowledge of performance) or tells them whether the production was correct or not (i.e., provides knowledge of results). Where such procedures

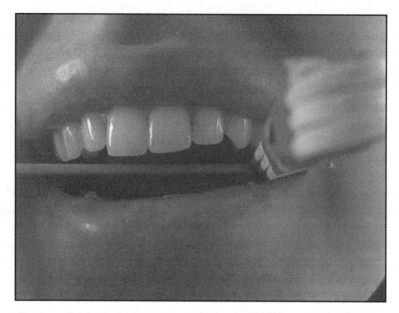

Figure 6–1. Example of a bite block created by taping three tongue depressors together. Photo courtesy of Stephen Sacks. Reprinted with permission. All Rights Reserved.

fail, the typical clinical response is to try a different procedure. Thankfully, there are many such procedures available even for /r/, and in most cases, one or more of these procedures will enable the client to generate a correct /r/.

Where these approaches are not being successful, one or more of the approaches discussed in Chapters 8 through 11 might be considered. Note that each of those approaches may have some approach-specific instructions and/or cuing strategies. It should be noted, however, that these alternative feedback approaches are unlikely to solve the problem by themselves. They must be integrated into a systematic program such as traditional articulation therapy or speech motor chaining. The feedback those approaches provide will ultimately need to be faded out so the child can produce the target sound without them; stabilize its production in syllables, words, and sentences; and then generalize correct production to everyday speech.

INTRODUCING SELF-MONITORING

A final suggestion for potentially increasing our success with traditional therapy is the use of self-monitoring. As noted previously, Van Riper implied that the earlier the child was made aware of and could recognize the errors in their own speech, the better the outcomes. In the previously discussed 1986 study by Koegel, Koegel, and Ingham, for children not yet generalizing to conversational speech, such generalization began shortly after self-monitoring was introduced. Note that Van Riper was likely dealing mostly with older children during his time, as universal school-based mandates were not introduced until the 1970s. Children over age 7 years are often quite aware that their speech is problematic, but they may not be able to identify their errors on a moment-to-moment basis. Thus, for this group, it makes sense to introduce self-monitoring as soon as possible (at least as soon as they have progressed to the phrase or sentence level). Trying to teach self-monitoring to preschool children is likely to be very difficult.

SUMMARY

Traditional articulation therapy as currently practiced appears to differ from its original form. Likewise, there is evidence that some aspects of traditional therapy may not work as advertised. It is conceivable that some of our difficulty with treatment success with this approach may, at least in part, reflect the fact that one or more critical components may not always be necessary. A modified therapy sequence (see Table 6–2) incorporating that evidence was proposed along with the principles of motor learning discussed in Chapter 5. The advantages of such modifications are that unlike some of the options presented in later chapters, (a) they are essentially free, and (b) their use is not limited to any particular tongue shape. A significant disadvantage is that these modifications may not be motivating enough for some therapy-resistant clients (i.e., those who have already experienced limited success with traditional therapy).

The chapters that follow represent more recent (and more extensive) attempts to change traditional therapy to make it more efficacious. Chapter 7 explores modifications to the approach itself, specifically changes to the sequence and/or the stimuli. Chapters 8 through 11 explore supplementing therapy with different forms of feedback for the client to maximize the establishment phase of therapy.

APPENDIX 6–1

Procedures for Establishing /r/ in Isolation

SPECIFIC ELICITATION APPROACHES

Shaping /ɝ/ from /l/ (Shriberg, 1975)

Here is a procedure for evoking a good retroflex /ɝ/ from a child who is unable to produce that sound. Once you have /ɝ/ established, you can teach the child to use a shortened version for consonantal /r/.

Phase	Instruction	Progression Criteria
Basic mobility	"Stick your tongue out"	Three consecutive correct
	"Stick your tongue out and touch the tip with your finger"	Three consecutive correct
	"Put your finger on the bumpy place right behind your top teeth"	Three consecutive correct
	"Put your tongue tip on the bumpy place"	Three consecutive correct
	"Put your tongue tip on the bumpy place and say /l/"	Three consecutive correct
	"Say /l/ and hold it until I say stop"	Five consecutive correct
Evoke /ɝ/	"Say /l/ and hold it, but while you hold it, drag the tip of your tongue slowly back along the roof of your mouth until the tip has to drop"	Five consecutive correct
(If unsuccessful)	"Let's practice pulling the tip of your tongue along the roof of your mouth. Pretend you are licking whipped cream off the roof of your mouth. Do it without making any sound."	Three consecutive correct (then return to previous step)

Shaping /r/ from /ð/ (Bleile, 2018)

Here the goal is a retroflex /r/. The child is asked to place their tongue as they would for producing /ð/. Then they are asked to begin producing /ð/ but quickly pull the tip of the tongue slightly up and back. The net result should be [r].

Shaping /r/ from /ɑ/ (Bleile, 2018)

Again, a retroflex /r/ is the target. Two variations are mentioned here. In both cases, if the child appears to be rounding their lips, they should be reminded to keep the lips pulled back slightly.

Variation One

Here the child is instructed to sweep the tongue tip along the roof of the mouth while saying /ɑ/. Then tell them to stop, while continuing to vocalize, and then drop the tongue tip slightly. The net result should be [r].

Variation Two

In this case, the child should produce a prolonged /ɑ/. While this is ongoing, ask them to raise the tongue tip and curl it back. The sound should change to [r].

SATPAC Approach to Eliciting a Good /r/[1]

Here the goal is a bunched /r/.

1. Ask the child to open their mouth while looking in a mirror. Keep it open and say /i/. The tongue should widen out. Then have them close the mouth halfway and repeat /i/. That should stabilize the tongue on the back molars.

2. Have them open the mouth fully and then close the mouth slightly to that /i/ with the mouth half open. Repeat several times. See if they are able to consistently reach that middle stabilized jaw position, while also helping to get that middle, widened out tongue.

3. (This step is required only for children who cannot consistently move from an open mouth to the mouth half open /i/.) Use the following steps to teach jaw grading. This procedure tunes them

---

[1]*Source:* Sacks, S. (2020, personal communication).

in to internal feedback so they learn what various levels of mouth opening feel like.

a. Start with teeth closed but smiling to show teeth (Position 1).

b. Then have them bite on a flat tongue depressor to achieve a teeth slightly open position (Position 2).

c. Then have them bite on a tongue depressor standing up on edge to achieve a wider (but not fully) open position—this is likely the best position for /r/ (Position 3).

d. Then have them make the mouth wide open (Position 4).

e. Randomly have them put the jaw into each of the four positions while looking in the mirror.

f. Practice many times in a session (can have parents do this with them at home).

g. Next session—repeat the random numbers to check accuracy. Then take away the mirror and let them use kinesthetic feedback. Ask them to close their eyes and then check in the mirror if they get it. Then take away the mirror. If they do not get it, repeat the practice with the tongue depressor. Then try it without.

4. Assuming they can achieve consistent jaw grading (whether spontaneously or after training from Step 3), evoke /r/ using jaw stabilization. This is done by taping three flat tongue depressors together and having them bite on them at one side of the mouth. You hold a second tongue depressor flat under the tongue and have them smile and say /i/ /i/, /irgæ/.[2] As they get to /irgæ/, you push back very slightly. Note: only push very slightly. The actual distance to be traveled is not very far. The positioning of the tongue depressors is shown in Figure 6–1.

5. Once established, the tongue depressors are removed stepwise (first the single one and then the three taped together), and the /irgæ/ is practiced many times on its own. Eventually they should be producing this facilitating nonsense form without any support.

6. For children with high palatal vaults, raising the back of the tongue all the way back to the top of the palate may be too difficult. In such cases, the better facilitating context might be /irʃæ/ or possibly /irdæ/. You may need to try both.

7. Once a good /r/ in the facilitating syllable is achieved, repeat many times.

---

[2]This context creates a dynamic movement between two different vowels and different consonant positions.

CUES FOR SPECIFIC COMPONENTS OF /R/ PRODUCTION[3]

1. Cues/instructions related to making the oral constriction:

   "Lift the front of the tongue up off the floor of your mouth."

   "Point your tongue tip toward the top of your head."

   "Try pointing the front part of your tongue at the bump behind your teeth."

   "Make sure the front part of your tongue is raised up near the roof of your mouth."

2. Cues/instructions related to tongue root retraction:

   "Try to make the back part of your tongue go back, like for /ɑ/."

   "Focus on pulling your tongue root straight back, not back and up" (if producing velar or uvular fricative).

   [If too far back] "Don't pull your tongue so far back that it feels unnatural."

   "Pretend you are holding a marble in between your tongue and the back of your throat."

3. Cues/instructions related to lateral tongue bracing:

   "Try to make the sides of your tongue go up for a butterfly bite."

   "Try to keep the middle of your tongue low, so there is a groove down the middle."

   "Push the sides of your tongue toward your top molars."

   "Bite gently on back side edges of your tongue with your back teeth."

4. Cues/instructions related to jaw aperture:

   "Focus on making your mouth/tongue feel tight."

   [If too clenched] "Open your mouth up a little bit more to let the sound out."

5. Cues/instructions related to appropriate degree of lip constriction:

   "Try tightening your lip corners a bit while you say the /r/ sound. Your lips should make a square shape."

---

[3]*Sources:* McAllister et al. (2020); Preston and Leece (2019).

CHAPTER 7

Treatment Option 2: Modifying Traditional Articulation Therapy

aving defined what traditional articulation therapy is and how it might be fine-tuned to make it more efficacious, we now turn to a second treatment option. In this case the goal is to make some more significant modifications to motor-based therapy. There are two possible ways to do this: The first involves the somewhat radical notion of randomly reordering the treatment sequence. The second largely retains the typical sequence but involves a much more extensive use of nonsense material and facilitating contexts.

CONCURRENT TREATMENT

A core aspect of traditional articulation therapy (and many treatments for speech sound disorders) is the now well-known treatment hierarchy. The sound is first taught in isolation (what Van Riper called establishment), then it is practiced in successively more complex linguistic contexts (Van Riper's stabilization step) including syllables, then words, then phrases, and finally sentences. Then the focus shifts to generalization to everyday situations including conversation. As discussed in Chapter 6, there are the added dimensions of imitation followed by spontaneous productions and different word positions. In this classic, bottom-up view (also called *reductionism* by some), the idea is to begin with the target skill at the most simple level, the speech sound in isolation, and then make the task progressively harder by embedding the sound in ever longer and ever more complex motor contexts. Moving up to the next level means that both the motor planning and the required movements will become ever more challenging. The presumption is that imitation is easier than spontaneous production, and some word positions may be easier than others. In the case of /r/, it is also assumed that stressed vocalic /ɝ/ is easier to learn than unstressed /ɚ/, which is easier to learn than consonantal /r/.

Intuitively, the bottom-up approach makes sense. Start simple and slowly make it harder. As discussed in Chapter 6, there is certainly evidence that traditional articulation therapy can work as originally outlined. However, like so much of traditional therapy, there has been limited evaluation about whether this rigid and gradual progression from shorter to longer linguistic contexts, imitation to spontaneous, and treating each word position separately is the most efficacious approach. There is some evidence that doing the reverse (i.e., using a totally top-down approach; see Camarata, 2021, as well as Hoffman & Norris, 2010) can also work. Although those approaches do not appear to be appropriate for treating single sound errors (see Preface herein), the fact that they may work in some other situations suggests that perhaps there is nothing magical about the standard easier-to-harder sequence. Empirical evidence emerging from studies by Steven Skelton and his collaborators suggests that completely randomizing the typical sequence may be at least as efficacious as following the typical sequence.

Skelton's approach is called *concurrent treatment* and like traditional therapy begins with establishment of the sound using whatever elicitation procedures are required. The major variation from traditional therapy occurs in the stabilization phase. Skelton and colleagues propose what to most will seem like a very radical idea: randomizing the sequence. An example of a randomized sequence for /r/ is shown in Table 7–1. The steps (tasks) listed are based on those in Table 6–1. Several items in Table 7–1 (noted with superscript "b") are steps that could potentially be eliminated, because our analysis of the evidence relating to traditional articulation therapy in Chapter 6 suggested that imitation above the syllable level may not be necessary for even the traditional sequence.

I must confess that the first time I saw such a list my initial reaction was something like "this is madness" or "this can't possibly work."[1] As with following developmental logic for choosing goals, following the typical easier-to-harder sequence makes so much intuitive sense. Why would we deviate from it? Two reasons come to mind. First, as noted there is not much specific evidence that the typical sequence is the best sequence.

---

[1]Steve Skelton has confessed in personal communication that he initially sought to confirm the need for the traditional sequence and assumed that such randomization would not work at all. He was also shocked that it worked.

Table 7–1. Example of a Randomized Treatment Sequence for /r/

Original Step Number[a]	Target
11	Spontaneous trials in single words—initial /ɝ/
33	Spontaneous trials in single sentences—final /ɚ/
25	Spontaneous trials in two- to four-word phrases—final /r/
6[b]	Imitative trials in single words—initial /ɝ/
5	Imitative trials in single syllables—final /r/
16[b]	Imitative trials in two- to four-word phrases—initial /ɝ/
20[b]	Imitative trials in two- to four-word phrases—final /r/
35	Spontaneous trials in single sentences—final /r/
15	Spontaneous trials in single words—final /r/
7[b]	Imitative trials in single words—final /ɝ/
13	Spontaneous trials in single words—final /ɚ/
36	Spontaneous conversation—all forms of /r/
12	Spontaneous trials in single words—final /ɝ/
14	Spontaneous trials in single words—initial /r/
29[b]	Imitative trials in single sentences—initial /r/
21	Spontaneous trials in two- to four-word phrases—initial /ɝ/
3	Imitative trials in disyllables—final /ɚ/
10[b]	Imitative trials in single words—final /r/
22	Spontaneous trials in two- to four-word phrases—final /ɝ/
30[b]	Imitative trials in single sentences—final /r/
8[b]	Imitative trials in single words—final /ɚ/
18[b]	Imitative trials in two- to four-word phrases—final /ɚ/
23	Spontaneous trials in two- to four-word phrases—final /ɚ/
19[b]	Imitative trials in two- to four-word phrases—initial /r/
17[b]	Imitative trials in two- to four-word phrases—final /ɝ/
32	Spontaneous trials in single sentences—final /ɝ/
27[b]	Imitative trials in single sentences—final /ɝ/
34	Spontaneous trials in single sentences—initial /r/

continues

Table 7–1. *continued*

Original Step Number[a]	Target
1	Imitative trials in single syllables—initial /ɝ/
24	Spontaneous trials in two- to four-word phrases—initial /r/
31	Spontaneous trials in single sentences—initial /ɝ/
4	Imitative trials in single syllables—initial /r/
9[b]	Imitative trials in single words—initial /r/
28[b]	Imitative trials in single sentences—final /ɚ/
2	Imitative trials in single syllables—final /ɝ/
26[b]	Imitative trials in single sentences—initial /ɝ/

Note. Adapted from "Concurrent Task Sequencing in Single-Phoneme Phonologic Treatment and Generalization," by S. L. Skelton, 2004, *Journal of Communication Disorders*, *37*, Table 4, p. 139 (https://doi.org/10.1016/j.jcomdis.2003.08.002).

[a]Relative to Table 6–1 herein.

[b]Step could be eliminated as they represent imitation above the syllable level (see Box 6–1).

It is simply what has always been done. Perhaps another way would be more effective? Second, and perhaps most powerfully, if what we are currently doing is not working so well, maybe shaking things up is at least worth a try for those clients where progress has stalled.

When using concurrent treatment, the child is first taught to produce the sound in isolation. Then the randomized sequence is introduced. Initially the child is given only one trial for each task on the list. If the production was correct, the next task on the list is presented. If the production is not correct, the child is given feedback and allowed to make another attempt. Regardless of whether the second attempt was correct or not, the next task of the list is then presented. Once the clinician reaches the bottom of the task list, if session time permits, practice continues back at the top of the list. Skelton (personal communication) indicated that in the 2004 study, on average, participants completed the list of tasks 1.65 times per 30-min session.

Evidence for Concurrent Treatment

To date, Skelton and his collaborators have presented a growing body of evidence in support of this approach. Four studies include data presented at professional conferences[2] (Skelton & Kerber, 2005; Skelton & Price, 2006; Skelton & Resciniti, 2009; Skelton & Snell, 2014), and another four were published in peer-reviewed journals (Skelton, 2004; Skelton & Funk, 2004; Skelton & Hagopian, 2014; Skelton & Richard, 2016). All eight studies are highlighted chronologically in Table 7–2.

Note that the studies in Table 7–2 reflect different populations, different study designs, and different speech sound targets. In all cases, experimental control was maintained, and significant improvement was noted. Experimental control was demonstrated in different ways. With the studies that used single subject designs (multiple baselines, alternating treatments), change did not occur until treatment was introduced for each participant. With the AB designs, the results were repeated over multiple participants. With the most recent study (Skelton & Richard, 2016), there was a control group that did not receive treatment. Some of the control group improved, but the experimental (treatment) group improved to a much greater extent. Thus, with all three types of studies, the change (or the greater degree of change) that was observed appeared to be the direct result of the treatment being provided.

There was some variation in the improvement observed in the studies in Table 7–2. The smallest amount of change occurred in the Skelton and Funk (2004) study, which was one of the studies with the weakest research design (Level IIb; see Table 1–2) and included the fewest details about the treatment that had been provided. In addition to being both the only group design and the highest level of evidence, the Skelton and Richard (2016) study is worthy of our attention for several additional reasons. First, it included /r/ as a target, making it most relevant for our focus here. Second, the treatment was being provided by the speech-language pathologists (SLPs) serving the children's schools and not the investigators. This strongly suggests that this approach is workable for SLPs practicing in the public schools. Finally, it is also worth noting that although the control group improved significantly less than the treatment group, some of the control group still showed some improvement. This is consistent with the idea that some of these children with persistent and residual errors will simply improve on their own (Flipsen, 2015) and supports our need for controlled studies such as these.

Clearly, the evidence is still limited and consists largely of small sample studies. More exploration is needed, but these findings suggest that concurrent treatment may work and should be seriously considered. Perhaps a more important question is whether a randomized treatment order is any more efficient than the conventional order. This is as yet uncertain. Only one study to date (Skelton & Price, 2006) appears to have involved such a direct comparison and suggests the randomized order may be superior. It included two 5-year-old children with one being treated for

---

[2]Conference presentations are usually only subject to minimal peer review.

Table 7–2. Summary of Evidence for Concurrent Treatment

Study (evidence level)	Population	Sample	Design	Tx Schedule	Tx Targets	Outcomes
Skelton, 2004 (Level IIa)[a]	7-year-olds with /s/ errors	n = 4 (three males, one female)	Multiple baselines across participants	Individual Tx 33–39 sessions 30 min each	/s/	All immediately improved from 0% to over 70% correct after Tx started; all maintained an average of 90%+ during Tx. All retained 80%+ correct at final posttreatment session.
Skelton and Funk, 2004 (Level IIb)[a,b]	4- to 6-year-olds with multiple errors	n = 3 (gender not specified)	AB design repeated across participants	Individual Tx No session details given	/k/ n = 1 /s/ n = 2	All immediately improved from 0% to over 45% correct after Tx started; all achieved 30%–50% correct in final conversation probe
Skelton and Kerber, 2005 (Level IIb)[b]	3;8–6;2 with multiple errors	n = 4 males	AB design repeated across participants with follow-up	Individual Tx; 35- to 40-min sessions	Four targets each with maximum differences	Three participants generalized to untreated targets
Skelton and Price, 2006 (Level IIa)	5-year-olds with multiple errors	n = 2 males	Alternating treatments design; one target = traditional order; one target = randomized order	Individual Tx; 35- to 40-min sessions	1 = /r, s/ 2 = /k, l/	1 demonstrated faster progress and better generalization with randomized (/s/) than traditional (/r/) 2 demonstrated progress and generalization similar on both orders

Study (evidence level)	Population	Sample	Design	Tx Schedule	Tx Targets	Outcomes
Skelton and Resciniti, 2009 (Level IIa)	4;2–5;10 with multiple errors	$n = 3$ males	Multiple baselines across participants	Individual Tx; 35- to 40-min sessions	/v, ʃ, θ, z/	Two children established all targets (third established all but /z/) Two children showed generalization across settings
Skelton and Snell, 2014 (Level IIa)	Children with childhood apraxia (age not specified)	$n = 3$ (gender not specified)	Multiple baselines across participants	Individual Tx; 40-min sessions	Individualized (CVC words)	All met goals and showed generalization to other untreated words
Skelton and Hagopian, 2014 (Level IIa)[a]	4- to 6-year-olds with childhood apraxia of speech	$n = 3$ (two males, one female)	Multiple baselines across participants	Individual Tx 12–28 sessions, 30 min each	/s, z, f, v/	All achieved 80%+ correct by the end of Tx; two of three achieved 90%+ correct in untreated words and phrases at end of Tx
Skelton and Richard, 2016 (Level Ib)[a]	6- to 9-year-olds with mild articulation errors	$n = 28$ (12 males, 16 females)	Group design; randomized controlled trial Experimental group $n = 16$, control group $n = 12$	Group Tx (four per group); 20 weeks of Tx, two times 30 min per week	/k, r, s, z, ʃ/	Significantly greater gain scores in experimental group (61% gain) compared to control group (26% gain)

Note. Tx = treatment.

[a]Peer-reviewed journal publication. [b]An AB design with only one participant is a case study and would normally be Level III. However, it was repeated over three participants which provides some degree of experimental control, making it Level IIb.

/s, r/ and the other being treated for /k, l/. For each child, one target was treated with the traditional order and the other target was treated with the randomized order. Findings for one child indicated faster and greater success for the randomized order (targeting /s/) than for the traditional order (targeting /r/). There was also far more generalization to untreated words and a storytelling context for the randomized order. For the other child, both targets progressed at a similar pace, and generalization was also similar with both orders. One confounding factor in this study is that according to Skelton (2020, personal communication), the one child where /r/ was targeted had great difficulty establishing correct production of that sound. The findings for that child may, therefore, have reflected the procedures used to elicit the sound rather than the order of treatment per se. That being said, at worst, this would mean that concurrent and traditional treatment orders would yield similar outcomes. Clearly additional such comparisons are needed.

SATPAC[3]

The other approach to modifying traditional articulation therapy is the *Systematic Articulation Training Program Accessing Computers* (SATPAC) that was developed by Stephen Sacks. This approach follows the general outline of traditional articulation therapy with a few key modifications that reflect (a) much more extensive use of nonsense (i.e., nonword) material, and (b) the choice of specific facilitating contexts in the construction of those nonsense materials. The use of facilitating contexts draws on the early work on coarticulation by McDonald (1964). As noted previously, many clinicians do not use nonsense materials. When they are used, they tend to be only simple syllables such as CV or VC forms. Doing so is consistent with how Van Riper (1954) discussed these to serve as a small part of stabilizing the sound before moving to real words. With SATPAC, however, their use involves more complex versions (e.g., beetseek for /s/ or eargah for /r/). Such forms are then practiced extensively in lists with minimal changes from word to word to develop a consistently correct motor pattern. Once the motor pattern is consistent, it is then transferred through the phrase and sentence levels and in systematically modified forms to expand the motor contexts in which the sound is produced.

---

[3]*Disclosure:* Peter Flipsen Jr., the author of the current book, is a coauthor of several studies documenting the efficacy of the SATPAC approach. His involvement has been solely to assist with research design and reporting of the results. He does *not* have any financial interest in this program. He receives no royalties, no remuneration, and no nonfinancial benefits of any kind from the SATPAC program or from the SATPAC founder Stephen Sacks.

This all occurs before real words are introduced. The goal is to establish a strong new habit to overcome existing bad ones. Real words are introduced at the sentence level, and specific monitoring of generalization to conversation is included. As much as possible, productions are practiced at normal speaking rates to assist with generating automaticity. Slower rates, which are often used in therapy, are avoided unless required to help with transitions from one program level or list to another.

As with most motor-based programs, SATPAC requires correct production of the sound before the nonsense syllables are introduced. This may not be needed where the child is stimulable for the target. However, where the child is not stimulable, any available method including those discussed in Chapter 6 could be used. Given the focus on facilitating context, the establishment of a new sound in SATPAC is done using at least a CV or VC or even longer context (e.g., "eergah" which is a VCCV). This is illustrated in a procedure for eliciting /r/ that was developed as part of the SATPAC approach. It includes jaw stabilization procedures and is outlined in Appendix 6–1.

After the target sound is established, SATPAC includes three specific phases. The first phase (called Establishment) involves systematic practice of the target in a facilitating context nonsense word through seven steps where the linguistic context becomes progressively longer and prosodic variations (e.g., stress and rate variations) are added. Steps 6 and 7 of the Establishment phase incorporate real words mixed in with the nonsense words to begin the process of transfer to real speech.

The second phase (called Practice) involves production of the target in a hierarchy of six lists, where each contains the target in varied nonsense forms. Across the lists, the context of the nonsense word becomes less and less facilitating. This is meant to encourage automaticity and flexibility. The last step (List 6) also incorporates real words to begin the transition to everyday speech. Examples of some of the nonsense forms that are used are shown in Table 7–3.

Table 7–3. Examples of Nonsense Words for /r/ in Practice Phase of SATPAC

List	Nonsense Words				
1	/irgæ/	/irgʌ/	/irgo/	/irgʊ/	/irgu/
2	/irgæ/	/irhæ/	/irkæ/	/irlæ/	/irjæ/
3	/irgæ/	/irlo/	/irnu/	/irwi/	/irtʃɪ/
4	/irgæ/	/ɛrgæ/	/argæ/	/orgæ/	/urgæ/
5	/irji/	/arnɑ/	/orvo/	/urʃu/	/ɛrwɛ/

The third phase (called Generalization/Transfer) involves the introduction of real words with practice starting with the words by themselves, and then moves progressively into phrases, sentences, and conversation. Treatment sessions are intended to be short (perhaps 10 to 15 min each) but are meant to involve high rates of production practice. For example, in the Sacks, Flipsen, and Neils-Strunjas (2013) study, participants were attempting up to 200 trials in each 10-min session. The lone participant in the Flipsen and Sacks (2015) study was attempting up to 400 trials per 30-min session.

Homework is considered critical to SATPAC. As discussed in Chapter 5, parents should be asked to do "as much as they can but at least 5 to 10 min per day." Specifically, the materials going home should be those that had been used at one level below where you are working in therapy. This avoids having the child practicing errors, since they should have mastered that level. Sacks (personal communication) suggests recording digital examples for parents to play as good models (or for parents to at least know what is expected). For purposes of recording homework, the child is typically given a mechanical counter to record correct productions. The counter also assists the child in developing self-monitoring skills. The data can be reviewed at subsequent sessions and rewards offered for reaching certain criteria of number of correct productions. The value of such reinforcement was discussed in Chapter 6 regarding the evidence for traditional articulation therapy.

In addition to highly structured and careful progression of the steps in the program, three other factors need to be considered. First, the specific facilitating contexts may vary from one child to the next. Second, if a child has other errors, those sounds should not be part of the practice sets (at least initially) to avoid additional reinforcement of those errors. Finally, some other sounds (e.g., /w/ when working on /r/) would need to be avoided for a time as they might interfere with correct production of the target. Developing the specific stimuli while keeping track of all these factors would be a considerable challenge. The SATPAC software is designed to manage all these moving parts. It is an Internet-based software program (see https://satpac.com/) that considers these factors and generates a set of customized practice lists for every step to be used in therapy. Clinicians purchase access to the software.[4] Training videos and access to professional support are also available.

Evidence for SATPAC

Data are available from five empirical studies of SATPAC. One study (Sacks, 2017) focused on children with highly unintelligible speech. Four others

---

[4]The basic program cost per clinician is kept reasonable so that it would be affordable for even public school clinicians as it could be used with multiple children.

focused on older children with residual or persistent errors; the latter four are highlighted chronologically in Table 7–4.

Two studies in Table 7–4 targeted /s/, and the other two targeted /r/. Three of the four studies were group designs, and the fourth was a case study. In all four studies, significant improvement was noted with the majority being remediated in 2.5 to 7.5 hr of direct therapy. Outcomes were maintained 6 to 24 months later. It should be pointed out that in two of the four studies (Flipsen & Sacks, 2015; Sacks et al., 2013), Stephen Sacks, the developer of SATPAC, provided all of the treatment. In the Flipsen and Sacks (2017) study, a second clinician was trained in the approach and provided treatment to half of the participants. In the Sacks and Flipsen (2013) study, two other clinicians were trained to provide all the treatment. Results obtained for all four studies were similar, suggesting that outcomes are generalizable beyond a single expert clinician.

As with concurrent therapy, the evidence for the efficacy of SATPAC is somewhat limited, and further study is indicated. Taken together, however, these findings suggest that SATPAC can be effective at remediating speech sound errors and should be given consideration as an alternative to traditional articulation therapy.

SUMMARY

Both concurrent treatment and SATPAC represent significant alternative forms of traditional articulation therapy that appear to be effective for remediating /r/ errors.

The relative advantages of concurrent treatment are that unlike some other options discussed in this book, (a) there are no costs involved, and (b) its use is not limited to any particular tongue shape. One notable disadvantage is that the random order suggested may be disconcerting for some clinicians or confusing for some clients.

SATPAC also has the advantage that its use is not limited to any particular tongue shape. As well, its extensive use of nonwords may be critical for some therapy-resistant clients to break their bad habits. An obvious disadvantage is the cost involved, which may be a barrier in some settings.

Clinicians choosing to use either concurrent therapy or the SATPAC approach would want to establish initial performance levels as a basis for monitoring progress and generalization. This might involve conducting a stimulability probe as shown in Appendix 4–1 and measuring accuracy in conversation using the form in Appendix 4–3. The word-level probe in Table 4–1 herein might also be worth administering. The particular words in that probe would then need to be excluded from therapy sessions.

In the chapters to follow, approaches are presented that involve providing the child with alternate feedback beyond the feedback they obtain from themselves and the verbal praise or correction we typically provide.

Table 7–4. Summary of Available Evidence for the SATPAC Approach

Study (evidence level)	Population	Sample	Design	Tx Schedule	Tx Targets	Outcomes
Sacks, Flipsen, and Neils-Strunjas, 2013[a] (Level IIa)	6- to 11-year-olds from two majority minority schools; many had other errors	n = 18 (11 males, 7 females)	Group design, quasi-randomized control trial[c] (delayed Tx control), one clinician	Individual sessions, 15 weeks at 10 min per week	/s/	Group 1 improved from 4% to 77% correct in conversation; averaged 59% 2 years later. Group 2 improved from 11% to 74% correct in conversation; averaged 81% 2 years later.
Sacks and Flipsen, 2013[b] (Level Ib)	6- to 8-year-olds with /s/ errors	n = 13 (7 males, 6 females)	Group design, randomized controlled trial (delayed Tx control), two clinicians	Individual sessions, 12 weeks at 15 min per week	/s/	Group 1 (Sacks as clinician) improved from 11% to 68% correct in conversation; Group 2 (second clinician) improved from 5% to 60% correct in conversation.
Flipsen and Sacks, 2015[a] (Level III)	12-year-old with a residual /r/ error, very stimulable	n = 1 male	Case study	Individual sessions, seven sessions at 30 min each	/r/	Improved from 0% to 90% correct in conversation 6 months later.
Flipsen and Sacks, 2017[b] (Level IIa)	7- to 9-year-olds	n = 6 (4 males, 2 females)	Group design, random assignment to two clinicians[d]	Individual sessions, 18–30 sessions at 15 min each	/r/	Improved from 25% to 94% correct in conversation 2 years later.

Note. Tx = treatment.

[a]Peer-reviewed publication. [b]Conference presentation. [c]Children in two schools: one school randomly treated first, then the other. [d]There was random assignment only to the two different clinicians (no other control, treatments identical).

While these approaches offer considerable promise, it should be noted that some children will simply not be able to relate to the alternate feedback being provided. In particular, children under age 6 years are unlikely to relate to any of them. Older children who have coexisting language or cognitive impairments may also have difficulty relating to such feedback.

CHAPTER 8

Treatment Option 3: Adding Supplemental Tactile Feedback

Having discussed traditional articulation therapy and a few modifications to its basic structure, we now turn our attention to a series of options for remediating /r/ that involve supplementing the feedback provided to the client. As mentioned earlier, these approaches are intended primarily to aid in the establishment of the correct target sound. The assumption is that these forms of alterative feedback will be the first step in some systematic therapy structure such as traditional articulation therapy and that the alternative feedback will eventually be faded out over time. The first of these feedback options (which represents our third treatment option overall) is the provision of alternative tactile feedback.

EXTERNAL VERSUS INTERNAL FEEDBACK

Feedback is received during speech either from outside sources (external) or from ourselves (internal). The discussion of feedback thus far has focused on external sources. In particular, in Chapter 5 external feedback was discussed in the context of the principles of motor learning. Specifically, it was discussed in terms of quantity (how much to provide), general type (knowledge of performance versus knowledge of results), and timing (how quickly to provide it). That discussion, however, presumed that the external feedback was verbal feedback provided by the clinician to the client. This is typical speech-language pathologist (SLP) therapy feedback.

It involves telling the client something. For example, in speech sound therapy we might say things such as "that was a good /r/" or "no, you forgot to keep your lips closed" or "did you mean one or run?" In later chapters, other forms of external feedback are discussed, but here the focus is on how to optimize internal feedback.

During speech, we receive internal feedback in several forms. We receive tactile feedback when one articulator contacts another. We receive kinesthetic feedback about the speed and direction of the movement of the articulators. We receive proprioceptive feedback about where the articulators are physically in space at any one moment in time. Finally, we receive auditory feedback (both air and bone conducted) about the acoustic output of the movements. Most of the time there is little or no conscious awareness of the internal feedback being received. In the process of providing external feedback to the client, one goal is to bring the internal feedback to the client's conscious attention. The principles discussed in Chapter 5 are partly intended to optimize that process. We begin with constant feedback on every attempt but wait a few seconds after each attempt before providing it. This allows the client to experience their own feedback. We initially provide specific information about what the client did or did not do correctly (knowledge of performance). This allows them to experiment with the movements or placements and experience both their own feedback and ours. We then slowly reduce the frequency of feedback and switch to only letting them know if their production was correct or not (knowledge of results). This allows them to begin making conscious decisions about what they need to be doing to consistently produce the correct target. This effectively is a form of self-monitoring instruction. We then extend this to encourage generalization by assigning homework that includes specific activities for monitoring their own speech outside of the therapy room.

When verbal feedback is provided, a few basic assumptions are implied. First, it is assumed the client is able to hear what is said; that is why there is always the concern about hearing status. Second, it is assumed that the client knows what is meant by the feedback, and that is why assessing language comprehension skills is so important. And third, it is assumed that they are able to use the feedback we provide together with their own internal feedback to make adjustments to what they are doing with their articulators.

However, despite the fact that the vast majority of children and adults with speech sound disorders have normal hearing acuity and normal language comprehension skills, not all of them seem to benefit equally from our verbal feedback. They are not able to use it to successfully correct their productions. One possible reason for this lack of success might be that even with the best and most appropriately structured verbal feedback, some clients may have limitations in the internal feedback that is available to them.

DIFFERENT KINDS OF INTERNAL FEEDBACK

As mentioned previously, internal feedback is continuously being received during speech. This includes auditory feedback (what you hear), proprioceptive and kinesthetic feedback (the sensation of where the articulators are and the speed and direction of their movements), and tactile feedback (the sensation of touch as one articulator contacts another). The focus in this chapter is on tactile feedback.

THE ROLE OF TACTILE FEEDBACK IN SPEECH

Despite considerable research and speculation, the precise role of tactile feedback in monitoring our own ongoing speech is still poorly understood. A number of studies, conducted mostly from the 1960s through the 1980s, offer some insight particularly relative to the production of /r/ that suggest some direction for therapy.

Tactile Sensitivity and /r/

As discussed in earlier chapters, when /r/ is being produced, contact between the tongue and the rest of the vocal tract appears to be limited. Contact may be made as the sides of the tongue dorsum brace against the upper molar teeth for a bunched /r/ or against the lower molar teeth for a retroflex /r/. That said, although the surface of the human tongue has lots of fast-acting mechanoreceptors that provide tactile feedback, they are not distributed evenly. There are more of these receptors in the front of the tongue compared to the back of the tongue and more in the middle of the tongue compared to the lateral edges (Ringel & Ewanowski, 1965; Trulsson & Essick, 1997). The net result is that given the location of tongue to teeth contact for /r/, even when accounting for tongue bracing, there may be limited available feedback.

Tactile Sensitivity in Individuals With Speech Sound Disorders

Is it possible that individuals with speech sound disorders have reduced sensitivity to whatever tactile feedback is available? Findings from studies using various tasks have yielded mixed results. One study by Fucci (1972) measured sensitivity to vibration in five adults who produced misarticulations (sounds not specified) and five adults with normal speech. Those who produced misarticulations required a higher amplitude of vibration before they noticed the vibrations on their tongues than typically speaking individuals. This suggested reduced tactile sensitivity. Other studies of tactile sensitivity have used oral-form recognition tasks. These tasks involve placing small objects in the mouth and then asking the person to either describe or identify the shape or decide if two consecutive shapes were the same or different shape or size. Some studies using these tasks have shown poorer skill in children with speech sound errors (Ringel et al., 1970; Speirs & Maktabi, 1990), while other studies found no differences (Arndt, Elbert, & Shelton, 1970; Hetrick & Sommers, 1988). Thus, as a group, it is not at all clear whether individuals with speech sound disorders receive reduced tactile feedback from the oral cavity.

Tactile Sensitivity in Individuals With /r/ Errors

The more important question for our current focus is whether there is something unique about individuals with /r/ errors. Perhaps, only this subgroup, has reduced tactile sensitivity. Findings from at least three studies suggest this may be the case. First, Weinberg, Liss, and Hillis (1970) tested a group of 34 older children (12 to 18 years old) with persistent /r/ errors who had been in therapy for at least 2 years. Findings indicated significantly poorer oral form recognition compared to a group of 35 normal-speaking peers.

A second study by McNutt (1977) used two measures of tactile sensitivity and three groups (15 each) of 12- to 15-year-old children. One group had no speech errors, one group had errors only on /s/, and the third group had errors only on /r/. On two-point discrimination (how close together two points could be before they are no longer recognized as being separate points), McNutt found that compared to the other groups, the children with /r/ errors required larger distances before they could recognize two separate points. This difference was observed at three different sites on their tongues. Likewise, on oral form recognition, the children with /r/ errors made significantly more recognition errors than the other two groups. Children with /s/ errors did not differ on either measure from the children with no errors.

A third study by Jordan, Hardy, and Morris (1978) included nine first-grade boys who scored outside the normal range on a single-word articulation test. All produced errors on /r/, and most also produced other errors. A control group included nine boys with no speech errors. Each boy was fitted with a custom artificial palate embedded with five contact sensors (similar to electropalatography [EPG] as described in Chapters 1 and 9 except with fewer sensors). Each sensor was connected via a tiny wire to a different colored light. The boys were trained to light up each color independently (i.e., to contact each sensor by itself). Two to three weeks later, they were brought back and the procedure was repeated, but this time a topical anesthetic was applied to the tongue before testing. Both groups were able to learn to do the task under both conditions. However, the children with speech errors required significantly more trials to learn the task under both conditions than their normal-speaking peers.

Together the findings from these three studies suggest the possibility that at least some children with /r/ errors have reduced oral tactile sensitivity. Assuming that is true, is it possible that providing supplemental oral tactile feedback might be the key to mastering /r/ for these children?

SUPPLEMENTING TACTILE INPUT

The notion of putting something in the mouth to assist with speech sound learning is not new. Clinicians have long been known to use tongue blades, ice chips, or flavored cotton swabs to raise intraoral awareness or to demonstrate the correct placement for a sound. For children who substitute /t/ for /k/, it is not uncommon for clinicians to use a tongue depressor to hold down the tongue tip to force the back of the tongue to come up to the velum for correct closure for /k/. Recall also from Appendix 6–1 the use of tongue depressors (as bite-blocks) in the Systematic Articulation Training Program Accessing Computers (SATPAC) method for eliciting /r/. Like so much of what is done in traditional articulation therapy, however, there has been limited systematic validation of such procedures. Clinicians incorporate them but do not usually evaluate them in any systematic way (but see Ruscello, 1995b, for a discussion of some early attempts). They typically try one thing and see if it works for a particular client. If it does, that is great, but if it does not, they simply try something else.

The approaches discussed in the following sections all assume that supplemental tactile feedback may be key to remediation of speech errors for some children. In each case, the goal is to be more systematic in the development of specific tools or approaches to do so.

SUPPLEMENTAL TACTILE INPUT AS FEEDBACK

Recall from Chapter 5 (under principles of motor learning) that when SLPs provide their verbal feedback, they are either telling the client (a) whether or not they were placing or moving the articulators correctly (knowledge of performance [KP]) or (b) whether or not the speech target was produced correctly (knowledge of results [KR]). It was also noted that the available evidence suggests that therapy should likely start with providing KP and then slowly switch to providing KR. Making this change allows the client to become their own therapist by combining the KR feedback with the feedback they receive from their own articulators and what they hear.

With supplemental tactile feedback, the client is effectively receiving KP. They learn more about what the articulators are doing. To be consistent with principles of motor learning, the tactile feedback must therefore be faded out over time to allow this switch to using their own feedback to take place. The idea that tactile feedback will not automatically generalize to speech without that supplemental feedback is also supported by a number of studies of other kinds of supplemental feedback (e.g., Fletcher et al., 1991; Gibbon & Paterson, 2006; McAlister Byun & Hitchcock, 2012; McAllister Byun, Hitchcock, & Swartz, 2014).

Box 8–1

Alternative feedback is intended largely for the establishment phase of therapy.

As therapy progresses to stabilization and generalization, the new feedback must be faded out.

SPEECH BUDDIES

An SLP and an engineer walk into a bar. Although it sounds like the opening line to a joke, it loosely describes how one approach to providing supplemental tactile feedback for speech sound intervention was born. Gordy Rogers (the SLP) and Alexey Salamini (the engineer) were good friends in high school who continued close contact through college and beyond. At some point after graduate school, they met up, and (as friends often do) they were sharing work stories. As they tell it, Rogers was lamenting his challenges with helping some of his clients achieve correct placement and movement for speech sounds. Salamini suggested that technology might be able to help. Perhaps they could come up with a device or a set of devices to place in the mouth to assist, and the idea for Speech Buddies was born (Rogers, personal communication, 2011).

Rogers and Salamini immediately saw the possibility of such devices both as a way to assist other SLPS and as a business opportunity. To create a viable business, they also knew they would have to be much more systematic in their approach. They fine-tuned their designs and worked with some manufacturers to develop a consistent process to build them. They then registered Speech Buddies as Class I medical devices with the U.S. Food and Drug Administration (FDA).[1] They ended up creating five

---

[1]Being registered is not the same as being approved. Registered simply means that the FDA has reviewed the manufacturing procedures and determined that these devices are

separate devices (one each for /s/, /ʃ/, /tʃ/, /l/, and /r/). They are available both individually and as a set. The Speech Buddies for /s/ and /r/ are shown in Figure 8–1.

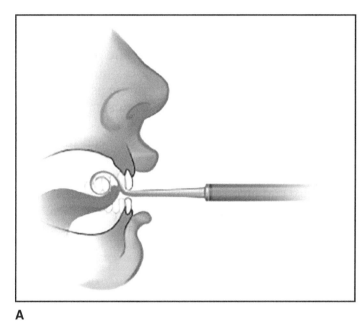

A

Figure 8–1. A. Speech Buddies tool for /r/. **B.** Tool for /s/. Both are in their intended positions within the mouth. Copyright 2020 Speech Buddies, Inc. Reprinted with permission. All Rights Reserved.

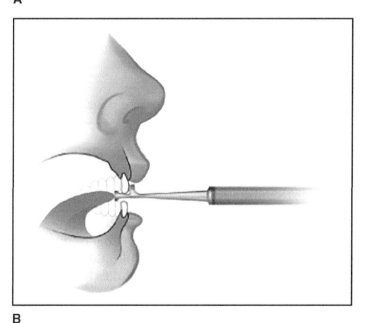

B

physically safe to put in a child's mouth. It does not mean that the FDA says they will actually improve speech. Class I medical devices are low-risk devices, and this category also includes such things as bandages, crutches, and nonelectric wheelchairs.

Each device has a handle that is initially held by the clinician. This may eventually be held by a parent, speech assistant, or the child themselves. The opposite end is placed in the mouth and held by the teeth at a dental stop (a specific site on the device where it rests against the teeth) to ensure correct positioning.[2] This effectively provides a specific location for tongue placement to begin the process of learning to correctly produce the sound.

Prior to starting therapy, a baseline probe should be recorded to serve as the basis for monitoring progress and generalization. This might involve conducting a stimulability probe as in shown in Appendix 4–1 and measuring accuracy in conversation using the form in Appendix 4–3. The word-level probe in Table 4–1 might also be administered. The particular words in that probe would then need to be excluded from therapy sessions.

Following the collection of baseline data, the client is introduced to the device and given an opportunity to attempt the target sound. The idea is that once the tongue is in the right place, the clinician provides specific instructions on how to produce the sound. Once correct production is established, the use of the device is faded out to assist with stabilization and generalization of the sound.

As can be seen in Figure 8–1, the /r/ device is coil shaped. The client is instructed to use the tip of their tongue to unroll the coil while attempting to say the sound. In so doing, the tongue tip curls back on itself yielding a retroflex /r/. This device was designed with that shape in mind. More information on the devices including videos demonstrating their use can be found at their website (https://www.speechbuddy.com/).[3]

EVIDENCE FOR SPEECH BUDDIES

As with the developers of some of the other approaches discussed previously (Concurrent Treatment, SATPAC), the developers of Speech Buddies have attempted to document their efficacy through a series of treatment studies. At least six such studies were identified and are highlighted chronologically in Table 8–1.

Two of the studies in Table 8–1 (Rogers, 2013; Rogers & Chesin, 2013) represent peer-reviewed journal publications, and the other four are conference presentations. Four of the six studies included /r/ as a target for at least some participants. Five of the six studies were AB designs; several involved repetition of that design across multiple participants within the study.

---

[2]Interestingly, this also provides the benefits of jaw stabilization that were discussed in Chapter 6.

[3]Although not free, the Speech Buddies devices are relatively inexpensive.

Table 8–1. Summary of Available Evidence for Speech Buddies

Study (evidence level)	Population	Sample	Design	Tx Schedule	Tx Targets	Outcomes
Rogers, 2011 (Level III)	7;4	n = 1 male	AB design, parent-administered Tx	8 hr total Tx over 12 weeks	/s/	Accuracy in words and sentences improved from 20% to 98%.
Rogers, Lee, and Parmentier, 2012 (Level IIb)	4- to 16-year-olds; 8/12 also had language goals	n = 12 (5 males, 7 females)	AB design repeated across participants, Tx administered by five trained SLPs	Group sessions; average of 1 hr Tx per week (average total of 18 hr of Tx)	/s, ʃ, tʃ, l, r/	Accuracy in words and sentences improved from 23% to 83%.
Rogers and Chesin, 2013[a] (Level Ib)	5;0 to 8;11	n = 15 (6 males, 9 females)	Group design, random assignment, Tx administered by four trained SLPs Control group: traditional articulation Tx (n = 7; 3 males) Experimental group: traditional articulation Tx + Speech Buddy (n = 8; 3 males)	Eight, 25-min individual sessions	/s/	Experimental group accuracy in words improved from 0% to 74%. Control group accuracy in words improved from 2% to 45%. Significant difference in improvement between the groups.

continues

Table 8–1. *continued*

Study (evidence level)	Population	Sample	Design	Tx Schedule	Tx Targets	Outcomes
Cote, 2013 (Level III)	9;9 7 hr of previous Tx[b] Correct on word initial /r/ but 0% correct in other contexts	*n* = 1 female	AB design, author-administered Tx 7 hr of traditional Tx[b] + Speech Buddy	Weekly 30-min individual sessions	/r/	Accuracy immediately improved from 55% to 100% (in isolation) and from 43% to 80% (in words) with Speech Buddy in place. After treatment, word-level accuracy overall improved from 43% to 77% without Speech Buddy.
Rogers, 2013[a] (Level III)	8;10	*n* = 1 male	AB design, author-administered Tx	Eight, 25-min sessions over 7 weeks	/r/	Accuracy in words and sentences improved from 20% to 90%.
Heintz, 2015 (Level IIb)	Treatment-resistant school-age children (age not specified)	*n* = 20 (gender not specified)	AB design repeated across participants, Tx administered by multiple SLPs	At least eight Tx sessions (session length and format not specified)	/s, ʃ, tʃ, l, r/	Average accuracy in words across all targets overall improved from 29% to 79%. Average /r/ accuracy in words improved from 27% to 69%.

Note. SLP, speech-language pathologist; Tx = treatment.

[a]Published peer-reviewed study.

[b]Specific program was "Entire World of /r/" (Ristuccia, 2002).

152

All of the studies reported improvement with the use of Speech Buddies. The one group design (Rogers & Chesin, 2013) showed the clearest result with the addition of Speech Buddies to traditional articulation therapy, resulting in significantly greater gains than in the control group (traditional articulation therapy alone). The lowest level study (Cote, 2013; Level III) provided the most ambiguous result. There was a 43% improvement before adding in Speech Buddies, which was followed by a 34% (77 − 43) improvement after treating with the added Speech Buddies).

Taken together the available evidence suggests that Speech Buddies may be effective at remediating speech sound errors in general and /r/ in particular. Some of the studies involved therapy being administered by either parents or several different SLPs. This suggests that the effectiveness of these devices extends beyond the application by specific experts. As with many of the other approaches discussed in this book, the evidence base for Speech Buddies is still somewhat limited, and additional study is clearly needed.

REMOVABLE INTRAORAL APPLIANCE FOR /r/

Another device that has been proposed to assist with the tactile input was described in a study by Clark, Schwarz, and Blakeley (1993). This removable appliance was specifically designed to assist with /r/ remediation. The appliance was custom built for each speaker similar to a retainer or an EPG device (see Chapter 9). It hooked onto the molar teeth on each side and included an acrylic plate covering the palate. The description of the functional portion of the appliance was somewhat vague, but it appears to have had an additional block of acrylic sticking down from the posterior portion. This block likely served as a point of contact for the tongue; given its location, it would appear that a bunched /r/ was the intended target.

Clark and colleagues (1993) also included data from an efficacy study of the appliance. Thirty-six children (ages 8 to 12 years; 25 males, 11 females) participated. All had previously received at least 6 months of therapy for /r/ but had made no significant progress. Treatment for all participants involved presentation of specific word stimuli for practice along with whatever additional treatment their school-based clinicians chose to provide. Half of the participants (18/36) used the appliance, and half did not. Treatment was conducted in individual sessions of 15 min, twice per week for 6 weeks. Results indicated /r/ accuracy in words improved significantly more in the appliance group (from 6% to 52%) than in the no appliance group (from 5% to 24%). As with Speech Buddies, this suggested that the addition of the tactile feedback provided by the appliance helped improve /r/ production accuracy. Although at the time of publication (1993) the article listed the appliance as patent pending, as far as could be determined, no commercial product was ever made available for wider use.

SUMMARY

During normal production of /r/, there is likely minimal tactile feedback received from the articulators. This fact combined with the possibility that some children with /r/ errors may have reduced tactile sensitivity in the mouth suggests that supplemental tactile input may assist with remediating /r/ for at least some individuals. Evidence is available from a number of studies suggesting that some approaches that provide supplemental tactile feedback can be used to successfully remediate /r/ errors.

Of the tactile feedback approaches discussed, Speech Buddies would appear to be the only viable (and evidence-based) option for most clinicians. Its advantages include that (a) the device provides a consistent placement structure that provides real-time feedback, and (b) once the target sound is established, the device can be sent home for additional practice. There are several disadvantages including (a) cost of the devices, though this is typically a one-time expense; (b) only retroflex /r/ can be targeted; and (c) some clients may have an aversion to having a foreign object in their mouths.

It should of course be remembered that although lacking evidence, the use of tongue depressors or flavored cotton swabs to provide tactile feedback would also not be an unreasonable other option. If nothing else, they offer a very low-cost alternative and may prove of some value.

In the final chapters, our attention turns to providing different forms of external feedback. If, as the old saying goes, a picture is worth a thousand words, perhaps providing some alternative form of visual feedback may help some of our clients change what they are doing. Three different forms of visual feedback are presented with the focus of the next chapter being EPG. This is followed in subsequent chapters by discussions of visual acoustic feedback and ultrasound feedback.

CHAPTER 9[1]

Treatment Option 4: Adding Visual Feedback via Electropalatography

The next set of treatment options involves providing alternative external feedback to remediate /r/ errors. If the verbal feedback we provide to our clients is insufficient to establish new ways of producing /r/, perhaps additional visual input will do the trick. At least three different forms of visual feedback have been developed, and each has evidence supporting its use. These will be presented in the chronological order of their development. First up in this chapter is our fourth overall treatment option—electropalatography (EPG).

THE ROLE OF VISUAL INPUT IN SPEECH ACQUISITION

Before discussing EPG, however, it is important to consider visual input in general. In everyday conversation, visual input can be very informative. For example, it provides information on whether the conversational partner understood our intended message as well as information about their emotional state. During the speech acquisition period, it does the same, and it can also provide some limited information about articulator placement and movement. Unfortunately, most speech sounds are not very

---

[1]If you have not already done so, it might useful to review the general information on feedback in the first few pages of Chapter 8.

visible from the outside, so it is unlikely that what we can see on the faces of others helps very much (except in the case of the most anterior sounds). This is especially true for /r/.

VISUAL INPUT AND TRADITIONAL THERAPY

Although we do not gain much about speech sound production from looking at the faces of others, visual input does appear to play a role in speech remediation. Clinicians often incorporate it into traditional articulation therapy in at least two different ways. First, phonetic placement procedures for eliciting target sounds may include pictures or diagrams to describe how the sound is normally produced, especially in terms of what structures are involved and where they should be placed. The Sounds of Speech app discussed in Chapter 6 (and similar digital options) also offers the possibility of showing the movements involved in producing particular speech sounds. Although Brumbaugh and Smit (2013) reported that 65% of clinicians use "verbal, pictured, or graphic cues" in therapy, specific evidence for the efficacy of such cues appears to be lacking.

A second way in which visual input can be incorporated into traditional therapy is through the use of mirrors. Although specific evidence of the efficacy of their use appears to be unavailable, anecdotal evidence suggests that mirrors are used. This suggests that some clinicians find them helpful. The author's personal experience is that some children do in fact benefit from looking in a mirror to assist in learning to physically produce speech sounds. However, there are at least two possible concerns with their use. First, some children do not appear to benefit and in fact may become frustrated with the use of mirrors. This is not surprising given the nature of the task. Imagine the last time you tried to do something in front of a mirror that you don't normally do. It can be quite difficult to get oriented to the movements because of the "mirror image" problem. Everything feels backward. Some children simply cannot get around that problem. The second concern with using mirrors relates specifically to /r/. Given that it is not an especially visible sound (except if attempted in an exaggerated way with the mouth wide open or to a limited extent with a retroflex /r/), mirrors may be of limited value.

POTENTIAL ADVANTAGES OF VISUAL FEEDBACK

Diagrams and mirrors aside, is it possible that some other form of visual feedback might assist with the remediation of /r/? In general, Hitchcock and Cabbage (2019) suggest several possible advantages for its use in speech remediation. First, the visual feedback supplements the external auditory feedback provided by the clinician and any internal feedback the client receives. Second, it may change the attentional focus from internal to external. As discussed in Chapter 5, an external focus (putting our attention onto something outside of ourselves) may be an advantage for some clients. Third, all three of the forms of visual feedback discussed here involve the use of some sort of instrumentation. For many clients, the instrumentation may raise their motivation to engage in therapy (i.e., the allure of technology and/or the cache of being able to "show off" to peers).

CHALLENGES OF PROVIDING VISUAL FEEDBACK

The mirror problem raised earlier highlights an important caveat that comes with providing supplemental visual input of any kind. Like typical verbal input, it is important that the client be able to understand the nature of the input and how to relate to it. Hitchcock and Cabbage (2019) suggested that ideal candidates for therapy involving supplemental visual input would have normal vision, have normal cognitive skills (i.e., be able to understand the images), and be able to sit and attend well. This would typically mean these approaches are best suited for children who are 7 years old and older. However, even clients who meet these criteria may not be able to benefit from these forms of visual feedback, and there is no clear way as of this writing to identify which clients will or will not benefit. The fact that approaches such as EPG have been used with some success with individuals with Down syndrome (e.g., Cleland et al., 2009) suggests that they should not immediately be ruled out even for individuals with cognitive impairments.

USE OF ELECTROPALATOGRAPHY AS FEEDBACK

Specific to EPG, more detail is provided later, but in general it provides the client with information about how the tongue contacts the palate. This is an alternative or supplement to the verbal feedback the speech-language pathologist provides about whether or not they were placing or moving the articulators correctly. In Chapter 5 in the discussion of principles of motor learning, knowing what the articulators are doing was referred to as knowledge of performance (KP) feedback. It was also noted that over time, KP feedback should change to knowledge of results (KR) feedback. Here the clinician simply tells the client whether or not the speech target was produced correctly. Doing so allows the client to eventually become their own therapist by combining the KR feedback with the feedback they receive from their own articulators and what they hear.

The EPG display provides the client with KP, because they see what the articulators are doing. They may also be receiving either KP or KR feedback from the clinician. To be consistent with principles of motor learning, both the visual feedback and any other KP feedback must therefore be faded out to allow the switch to using their own feedback to take place. This fading out would involve practice first with the device in place, then removing it for one or two trials and testing for generalization. As it is unlikely to be retained initially, the device would then be put back in for additional practice and feedback. Then slowly, practice without the device would be increased over time, and practice with the device in place would decrease. The idea that EPG feedback will not automatically generalize to speech without the EPG device in place is also supported by a number of studies of therapy using supplemental feedback (e.g., Fletcher et al., 1991; Gibbon & Paterson, 2006; McAlister Byun & Hitchcock, 2012; McAllister Byun et al., 2014).

Box 9–1

EPG feedback is intended largely for the establishment phase of therapy.

As therapy progresses to stabilization and generalization, the new feedback must be faded out.

BASICS OF EPG

Electropalatography involves the generation of images of tongue-to-palate contact that the client can then use to modify how they produce speech sounds. As discussed in Chapter 1, this idea of looking at tongue-to-palate contact dates back to at least the 1870s. About a hundred years later, technological developments would transform what were initially only static snapshots of a single tongue-to-palate contact event into a viable research tool for examining changes in tongue-to-palate contact across a few speech sounds. The interested reader may wish to revisit Chapter 1 for a discussion of the evolution of EPG.

In the last 20 years, advances in computing power and reductions in the cost of creating the required pseudopalates has meant that EPG has become a viable clinical tool in many contexts.[2] Clinicians and research-

---

[2]Cost may still be a barrier in some settings. As of this writing, the cost of construction of a custom pseudopalate varies from $300 to $600 and these can only be used with a single individual. There are also usually costs for access to the software.

ers are now able to observe how tongue-to-palate contact changes on a moment-to-moment basis across extended utterances.

Referring back to Figure 1–1, there are two functional components to an EPG system. The first is the pseudopalate that is custom constructed for each client by taking an impression of their upper teeth and palate. An example of a dental cast created by such an impression is shown in the rightmost portion of Figure 1–1. Using this cast, an EPG palate or pseudopalate is created that clips onto the teeth, an example of which is shown in the center portion of Figure 1–1. The pseudopalate follows the shape of the speaker's palate and contains a series of small pressure sensors. Each sensor is connected to a tiny wire, and the wires are bundled together and hang out of the mouth. These wire bundles are then connected to the second functional component of an EPG system, the computer display. The leftmost portion of Figure 1–1 shows a stylized version of such a display. Each square in the image corresponds to one of the pressure sensors in the mouth. The darkened squares indicate tongue-to-palate contact, and the white squares represent points of no contact. In the example in Figure 1–1, the speaker is producing a normal /s/ where the tongue seals off each side of the mouth on the teeth and forces air down the middle of the tongue and out the opening in the middle of the front teeth (the single white square in Row 1 of the image). This image provides the client with the visual feedback they use, along with clinician instructions, to modify their speech. More examples of pseudopalates and on-screen EPG images are shown in Figures 9–1 and 9–2.

Compare Figure 9–1 and Figure 9–2. Note the difference in the construction of the pseudopalates. More importantly, note the differences between Figures 9–1B and 9–2B. This illustrates the differences in the contact patterns for /s/ and /r/, respectively. It is the difference in these contact patterns that the client learns from.

Two additional elements may be available with some EPG systems. First, some manufacturers may provide a training palate (along with the pseudopalate). This has no sensors but can be used to allow the client to experience the presence of the pseudopalate by itself and acclimate to the modified oral sensations involved. This may be quite useful as some children have different levels of tolerance for the presence of anything foreign in their mouths (including a pseudopalate).

A second additional element available with some EPG systems is the possibility of a split-screen presentation. When available, a model of the target can be presented on one side of the screen that the client can then try to match in therapy. These may be prestored models, or they may be generated by the clinician who often has their own custom pseudopalate. In the absence of a split-screen setup, the clinician can print out a model in advance to be used as the client's target.

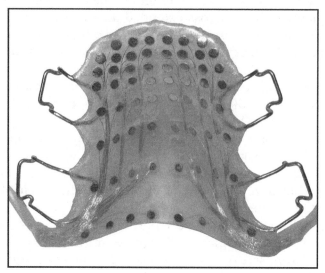

A

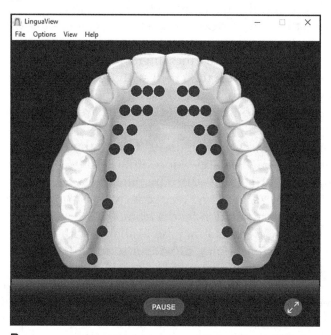

B

Figure 9–1. Electropalatography equipment from Rose Medical. **A.** A pseudopalate. **B.** An example of the on-screen image for the production of /s/. Copyright 2020 Rose Medical Solutions Ltd. Reprinted with permission. All Rights Reserved.

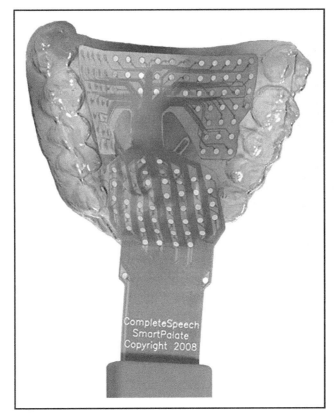

A

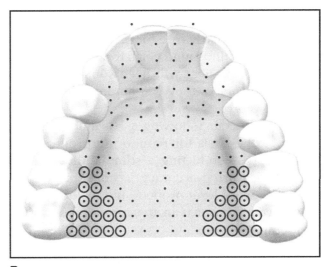

B

Figure 9–2. Electropalatography equipment from CompleteSpeech. **A.** A pseudopalate. **B.** An example of the on-screen image for the production of /r/. Copyright 2020 SmartPalate International. Reprinted with permission. All Rights Reserved.

Box 9–2: Consider the Teeth

Clinicians contemplating the use of EPG should be aware of the potential impact of dental changes. Children ages 6 to 12 years, the primary population being discussed in this book, are in a period of mixed dentition (i.e., they are in the process of losing their primary teeth that are then replaced by permanent teeth). If teeth are lost and/or replaced while EPG treatment is ongoing, the pseudopalate may no longer fit very well.

Some clinicians may be concerned about the presence of the pseudopalate affecting the quality of speech, but such concerns appear to be unwarranted. McLeod and Searl (2006) reported on a study of normal-speaking adults adjusting to the presence of a pseudopalate. Participants reported that their speech felt different, but listener judgments and acoustic analysis suggested minimal impact on speech output, especially after the first 1 to 2 hr of use.

Orientation to EPG

As with all clinical strategies, the client must be oriented to the equipment, the task requirements, the feedback being presented, and the overall arrangement. This is particularly true for unfamiliar technologies such as EPG, acoustic displays, or ultrasound. Such tools should never be assumed to be "plug and play." The client will need some time to be oriented to the system and its elements, or they will not be able to take advantage of what it has to offer.

Orientation would occur following a baseline probe that would be recorded to serve as the basis for monitoring progress and generalization. This might involve conducting a stimulability probe as shown in Appendix 4–1 and measuring accuracy in conversation using the form in Appendix 4–3. The word-level probe found in Table 4–1 might also be considered. The particular words in that probe would then need to be excluded from therapy sessions.

In the case of EPG, Hitchcock and Cabbage (2019) suggest that the first two treatment sessions be set aside strictly for orientation. An adaptation of their suggested outline for such an orientation is presented in Table 9–1.

Establishment and Stabilization With EPG

Carter and Edwards (2004) suggested a general outline to EPG therapy that might involve 8 to 10 sessions lasting about 30 min each. This would

Table 9–1. Possible Electropalatography Orientation Plan

Session 1	Review tongue anatomy
	Introduce the system
	Orient client to the image on the screen
	Have client try out the practice palatea
	Try out pseudopalate and phonetic placement cues for /r/
	Check client comprehension
	Send practice palate home[a,b]
Session 2	Attempt to match pseudopalate views—playing with the images of other sounds client can produce correctly
	Teach phonetic placement cues for /r/ while comparing their production to target image by clinician
	Check client comprehension

Note. Adapted from *Biofeedback for Childhood Speech Disorders: Practical Information for Clinicians* [Webinar], by E. R. Hitchcock and K. Cabbage, November 2019, presented to American Speech-Language-Hearing Association Special Interest Groups 1, 16, and 19; and "Efficacy of Electropalatography for Treating Misarticulations of /r/," by E. Hitchcock, T. McAllister Byun, M. Swartz, and R. Lazarus, 2017, *American Journal of Speech-Language Pathology, 26,* pp. 1141–1158 (https://doi.org/10.1044/2017_AJSLP-16-0122).
[a]If available.
[b]Client to wear 5 to 10 min per day for 1 week.

be followed by a move to generalization training without the device. EPG therapy would start with having the child copy the contact pattern for the target sound but not actually say the sound out loud. This gives them a chance to make associations between the movements in the mouth and changes on the screen without the distraction of their auditory output. This may require one to two sessions of practice. The next few sessions would involve practicing production of the target in isolation while viewing the feedback on the screen. Then a few sessions could be spent practicing the target in various word positions. Once this is stabilized, production could proceed to phrases and sentences. The last few of those would involve transitioning to practice without the device in place (i.e., systematically fading out the use of the device and the visual feedback).

Hitchcock and colleagues (2017) offer an alternative process for establishment and stabilization. They suggest that the first session after orientation begin with practice with the pseudopalate in producing two to three speech sounds that the client already produces correctly. An obvious advantage to this approach is early success to encourage the client's continued practice attempts. It can also be similar to free play and emphasizes that therapy can be enjoyable. Using a split-screen display, the client could attempt to match the clinician's productions of the known sounds on the screen. In their treatment study, Hitchcock and colleagues then proceeded to practice with /ɝ/ in isolation followed by initial /r/ in nonsense syllables (e.g., /rɑ/, /ri/, /ru/). A traditional hierarchy of practice (e.g., CV nonwords, CV real words, CVC nonwords, CVC real words, etc.) would follow. From the syllable level onward, the use of the pseudopalate (and the resulting visual feedback) would start to be faded out. Within each session, use of the pseudopalate would be reduced from 100% of trials (every trial) to 50% (every other trial) to 0% (no use) to encourage generalization to production without the device.

The generalization phase would begin once some preset level was reached. There is no solid evidence suggesting what that ideal point might be. One possibility is to use success at the real word level (e.g., 80% correct or higher) without the device. From this point onward, the pseudopalate would only be used on occasion to provide reminders if production accuracy became too low at higher levels in the treatment hierarchy.

Additional details about the application of EPG for speech sound disorders can also be found in Gibbon and Wood (2010).

EPG AS A REMEDIATION TOOL

There is an extensive list of papers and studies relating to the use of EPG for speech sound remediation. Its efficacy has been demonstrated with several different populations including individuals with hearing impairment, cleft palate, Down syndrome, cerebral palsy, and speech sound disorders without any obvious cause. The majority of the studies have been case studies, though a few somewhat larger samples have been used. In 2013 Fiona Gibbon compiled a bibliography listing much of this research. That bibliography is available online (https://pdfs.semanticscholar.org/6aa9/ad 6803435b5ed23a174309b434e13d14598d.pdf).

As it turns out, most of the treatment studies of EPG have focused on its use to remediate stops, fricatives, and affricates. Although some practicing clinicians who currently use EPG report doing so successfully for /r/, there is limited published empirical evidence to date relative to /r/. With limited contact between the tongue and the rest of the vocal tract during production of /r/, researchers may have assumed (as I did until recently) that EPG was of limited usefulness. However, looking at Figure 9–2B, some contact can be observed using EPG systems. Such contact patterns involve lateral tongue bracing against the upper molar teeth during attempts to produce a bunched /r/. Speakers whose optimal tongue shape is some other shape may be less likely to benefit from the feedback provided by EPG.

EVIDENCE FOR EPG AND REMEDIATION OF /r/ ERRORS

Although somewhat limited, there is in fact some published evidence that suggests that EPG may be useful for remediation of /r/ errors. Three specific studies could be identified, and these are highlighted chronologically in Table 9–2.

A review of Table 9–2 reveals mixed outcomes. In each case, /r/ was successfully remediated using EPG for some individuals but not for others. As suspected, this is likely because only a bunched /r/ would yield useful feedback when using EPG. For speakers where another tongue shape is more efficient, EPG may not provide much useful feedback. In their discussion of this approach, Hitchcock and colleagues (2017) state this quite explicitly noting that "EPG may be a less effective treatment for rhotic misarticulations . . . because it offers limited options for lingual exploration" (p. 1155).

SPECIFIC MANUFACTURERS OF EPG EQUIPMENT

Over the years, several different companies have attempted to develop commercially available EPG systems. At least three have successfully done so.

One of the first commercially available systems was produced by Pentax Medical, who previously manufactured them under the Kay Elemetrics brand. Unfortunately, their palatometer system was recently discontinued.

Rose Medical produces their LinguaGraph EPG system (details available at http://rose-medical.com/electropalatography.html). Images in Figure 9–1 represent Rose Medical equipment.

Finally, a company named CompleteSpeech currently makes what they call their SmartPalate system (details available at https://complete speech.com/smartpalate/). Images in Figure 9–2 represent CompleteSpeech equipment.

SUMMARY

The visual feedback provided by EPG may be the missing piece for some individuals with /r/ errors. There is some research evidence showing its efficacy. An obvious advantage to EPG is that it offers a somewhat direct view of what the tongue is doing inside the mouth. The feedback is also provided in real time. Disadvantages include (a) the costs involved, which may be a significant barrier; (b) it is limited to those for whom a bunched /r/ is the optimum tongue shape; (c) possible aversion by some clients

Table 9–2. Summary of Available Evidence for Use of Electropalatography (EPG) to Remediate /r/

Study (evidence level)	Population	Sample	Design	Epg System	Tx Schedule	Outcomes
Schmidt, 2007 (Level III)	7- to 12-year-olds	n = 9 with /r/ errors (8 males, 1 female) Five had other errors	Retrospective file review	Logometrix[a]	Two 30-min sessions per week 6–30 sessions each	5/9 mastered in Tx and generalized to spontaneous speech. 2/9 mastered in Tx but no follow-up data. 2/9 mastered in Tx but no generalization.
Fabus et al., 2015 (Level IIb)	9;5 to 10;1	n = 2 males where /r/ was treated	AB design repeated across participants	Complete speech	Weekly 45-min sessions for 10 weeks	One participant showed partial generalization 3 months later (accuracy 40%–100% across contexts). One participant 82% accurate at end of Tx but no follow-up data.
Hitchcock et al., 2017 (Level IIa)	6;10 to 9;10	n = 5 (2 males, 3 females)	Multiple baselines across participants	Complete speech	16 sessions	4/5 achieved correct production in treatment. 2/5 generalized to untreated words.

Note. Tx = treatment
[a]System appears to be no longer available.

to having something foreign placed in the mouth; and (d) the possibility that teeth changes may lead to the device not fitting well. The initial cost to the clinician to have their own device made to model productions may also be a barrier.

In the next chapter, we turn our attention to visual acoustic feedback.

CHAPTER 10[1]

Treatment Option 5: Adding Visual Acoustic Feedback

The fifth overall treatment option at our disposal is also the second form of visual feedback to be developed. This involves using visual acoustic feedback. A major potential advantage of this approach is its flexibility for the client relative to /r/ production. Unlike Speech Buddies that requires the client to produce a retroflex tongue shape or electropalatography (EPG) that may only be useful if the client attempts a bunched tongue shape, any tongue shape that yields a correct /r/ can be the target when using visual acoustic feedback. In fact, tongue shape itself may not actually have to be directly discussed (though it may be). A second potential advantage of visual acoustic feedback is that like EPG and ultrasound, the feedback can be available in real time (or with only a slight delay). A final advantage may be cost. Most readers will recall having learned about the basics of acoustic analysis in their undergraduate training either in a stand-alone acoustics course or as part of a phonetics or speech science class. Many may also recall being told at that time that routine clinical use of acoustic analysis was not feasible because of the need for expensive hardware and/or software. Cost and access to equipment, however, are no longer barriers. Although expensive systems are

---

[1]If you have not already done so, it might be useful to review the general information on feedback in the first few pages of Chapter 8 and information on visual feedback in particular in the first few pages of Chapter 9.

still available and continue to be used by researchers, inexpensive and/or free software is now available that can operate on the laptop computers that most clinicians already use.

A few important reminders are in order at this point. First, it is assumed that, if used, visual acoustic feedback by itself is not sufficient for successful speech sound remediation. The assumption is that it will be used as part of some systematic therapy structure such as traditional articulation therapy. Second, as with other alternative forms of feedback, its use is intended primarily as part of the establishment phase of therapy. Third, recall that Hitchcock and Cabbage (2019) suggest that ideal candidates for therapy involving any supplemental visual input should have normal vision, have normal cognitive skills (i.e., be able to understand the images), and be able to sit and attend well. This would typically mean visual acoustic feedback is best suited for children who are 7 years old and older. Cognitive skill level may be particularly important to remember given the somewhat abstract nature of the images the client is looking at with visual acoustic feedback.

VISUAL ACOUSTIC INPUT AS FEEDBACK

As mentioned in Chapter 5 (under principles of motor learning), when speech-language pathologists (SLPs) provide verbal feedback, they are doing so in one of two different ways. They are either telling the client (a) whether or not they were placing or moving the articulators correctly (knowledge of performance [KP]) or (b) whether or not the speech target matched the intended target (knowledge of results [KR]). It was also noted that the available evidence suggests that therapy should likely start with providing KP and then slowly switch to providing KR. Making this change allows the client to become their own therapist by combining the KR feedback with the feedback they receive from their own articulators and what they hear.

Visual acoustic feedback represents the output or product of the speech movements. As such, it represents KR. One might expect, therefore, that any learning that occurs should easily generalize. However, there are two reasons to suppose it would not do so easily. First, there is the abstract nature of visual acoustic feedback (discussed later). Second, studies of motor learning have shown that the frequency of feedback must be reduced over time. Otherwise, the client becomes too dependent on the feedback, and the skill being learned will not generalize. This explains why, like all other forms of feedback, visual acoustic feedback must be faded out to allow this switch to using their own feedback to take place.

Box 10–1

Reminder: Visual acoustic feedback is intended largely for the establishment phase of therapy.

As therapy progresses to stabilization and generalization, the new feedback must be faded out.

ATTENTIONAL FOCUS AND VISUAL ACOUSTIC FEEDBACK

Unlike the two other forms of visual feedback discussed in this book (EPG and ultrasound), visual acoustic feedback does not provide any direct information about what the tongue is doing. While EPG and ultrasound may force the client to simultaneously focus both externally (i.e., on the visual feedback) and internally (i.e., on what the tongue is doing), visual acoustic feedback on its own only requires the client to focus externally. This may be sufficient. Clinicians may simply advise the client to "make the peaks match the line on the screen." Alternatively, the clinician may add placement or shaping cues that focus the client internally at the same time. Recall from Chapter 5 that it is not clear whether an internal or external focus is the better approach. A study specific to /r/ by McAllister Byun, Swartz, Halpin, Szeredi, and Maas (2016) reported no clear advantage for either type of focus.

UNIQUE NATURE OF VISUAL ACOUSTIC FEEDBACK

Visual acoustic feedback is a very different kind of feedback. Unlike EPG feedback or ultrasound feedback (discussed in the next chapter), it does not show us directly what the tongue is doing. The image being seen represents a mathematical translation by a computer algorithm of the sound energy that was produced into an abstract image. It only indirectly illustrates what the speaker just did with their articulators. In order to use that feedback, the client must figure out how to move their articulators to change the on-screen image. That requires some amount of mental gymnastics for the client using this feedback. This reinforces the idea that this type of feedback is more appropriate for clients with sufficient cognitive abilities (i.e., those who are at least 7 years of age and have normal cognitive skills).

Despite its somewhat abstract nature and the need for some mental manipulation, there is evidence available (discussed later) demonstrating that visual acoustic feedback can be used to successfully remediate /r/ with some of our clients. Therefore, many of our clients will be able to take advantage of it.

ACOUSTIC INFORMATION CRITICAL FOR /r/

For many readers, it may have been some time since they studied acoustics, so a brief acoustics refresher is likely in order. In addition to the information presented here, the reader might wish to refer to Neel (2010) for additional information on clinical application of visual acoustic feedback.

As mentioned in Chapter 2, /r/ is a vowel-like sound involving only slight constriction within the vocal tract. It is also sometimes referred to as a resonant sound. As such, the dominant acoustic characteristics of this sound are the relative relationships among the sound frequencies being produced. Recall that voicing is generated at the larynx, and the sound source thus created contains a complex set of acoustic frequencies. This sound source is then filtered by the vocal tract (i.e., the resonating space above the larynx). The nature of the filtering is determined by the overall shape and configuration of the vocal tract. During this filtering process, certain frequencies stand out and other frequencies are deemphasized. The frequencies that stand out are known as the formant frequencies or formants; these are numbered in order such that the lowest frequency formant is referred to as F1, the next highest is F2, then F3, and so on.

The particular formants associated with each resonant sound depend on the location of the constrictions within the vocal tract. As many as five or six formants may be present, but most resonant sounds can be distinguished from other resonant sounds by specifying no more than F1, F2, and F3. Hitchcock and Cabbage (2019) note that F1 is usually determined by tongue height, F2 by tongue advancement (front to back location), and F3 by the points of maximal velocity within the vocal tract. For /r/, F3 is determined by a combination of the three known constrictions (lips, palate, pharynx). The specific frequencies for each formant vary from speaker to speaker because of differences in the length and configuration of each vocal tract, though values tend to be similar for individuals of the same age and sex.

TYPES OF VISUAL ACOUSTIC FEEDBACK

The acoustic product of the speech signal can be represented several different ways. Two methods are relevant to our discussion here, as they have been used successfully to remediate /r/.

Spectrogram Displays

The first and oldest method for visual acoustic feedback is the spectrogram display. An example of a wideband spectrogram (the most common form) is shown in Figure 10–1. Note that the display reveals frequency on the vertical axis and time on the horizontal axis. Intensity (or loudness) variations are shown by shades of gray with the loudest sound being the darkest. A white space indicates no detectable sound.

As indicated by the transcriptions along the bottom of Figure 10–1, four different nonwords are represented that illustrate the acoustic patterns for two glide consonants (/w, j/) and two liquid consonants (/r, l/). All four nonwords were produced by the same adult female speaker. In each case, you will notice five darker bands of energy. The lowest flat dark band along the very bottom represents the speaker's fundamental frequency (f0; the basic rate of vibration of the vocal folds). The other four bands represent the first four formants (from bottom to top: F1, F2, F3, F4). For our purposes, we can ignore F4.

Notice that unlike f0, which remains unchanged and thus is flat, the four formant bands all change in direction and extent as the speaker moves their articulators from the preceding vowel to the consonant to the following vowel. The rising and falling of the formants illustrates the changes in frequency as the constrictions in the vocal tract are changed. For example, in the first nonword (awa), F1 and F2 both drop very sharply from /ɑ/ to /w/ and then rise again very sharply from /w/ back to /ɑ/. At the same time, F3 rises slightly and then falls slightly afterward. Contrast that pattern with the third nonword (ara), where F1 falls only slightly from /ɑ/ to /r/ and then rises only slightly from /r/ back to /ɑ/. At the same time, F2 only just barely falls and then rises again afterward. Note, however, that F3 drops very sharply from /ɑ/ to /r/ and then rises sharply again as the speaker moves back to /ɑ/.

Relative to remediating /r/, recall that the classic substitution pattern is [w] for /r/. The key difference between /w/ and /r/ is what is happening with F2 and F3. For /w/, F2 and F3 go in opposite directions, while for /r/, F2 and F3 become very close together. This narrowing of the gap between F2 and F3 is the prototypical acoustic signature of American English /r/ (Boyce & Espy-Wilson, 1997: Kent, Dembowski, & Lass, 1996). As such, it is the key pattern that clinicians and clients must focus on when using visual acoustic feedback for remediating /r/. The SLP's goal would have the client do whatever is necessary to create this narrow distance between F2 and F3.

Linear Predictive Coding Spectrum Displays

Although spectrogram displays have been used successfully for remediating /r/ (e.g., Shuster et al., 1992, 1995), the display is somewhat crowded

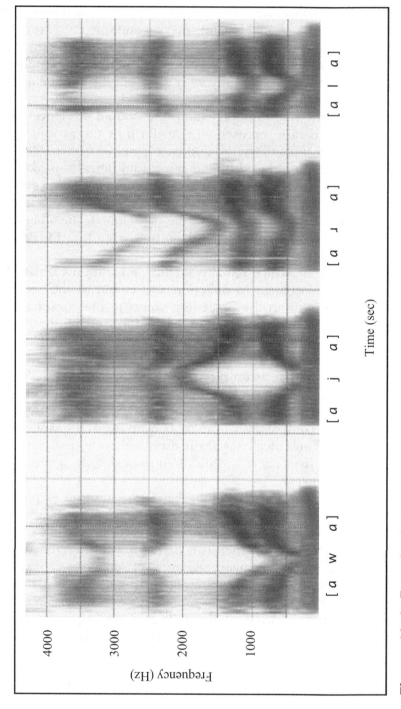

Figure 10–1. Example of wideband spectrogram for English approximant consonants in the nonwords awa, aya, aɾɑ, and ɑlɑ. From *Phonetic Science for Clinical Practice* (p. 179) by Kathy J. Jakielski and Christina E. Gildersleeve-Neumann. Copyright 2018 Plural Publishing. Reprinted with permission. All Rights Reserved.

and can be confusing for some clients even with some amount of orientation. Also, although real-time spectrograms can be generated quickly, there is a slight time delay. Given that the image represents frequency over time, the image represents a snapshot of what just happened, not what is currently happening. The second method for providing visual acoustic feedback for speech remediation gets around both of these shortcomings. This approach is the LPC (linear predictive coding) spectrum display. These displays show amplitude on the vertical axis and frequency on the horizontal axis; both variables in the display are changing in real time during speech production. Thus, they can be tracked with essentially no time delay. As a result of these advantages, LPC displays have been used in most recent studies of visual acoustic feedback for /r/ (e.g., Campbell & McAllister Byun, 2018). Figure 10–2 provides examples of LPC displays for a normal /w/ (Figure 10–2A), a normal /r/ (Figure 10–2B), and a derhotacized /r/ (Figure 10–2C).

The peaks shown in each panel of Figure 10–2 represent the formant frequencies for the three different productions. Each panel shows at least five formants, although as noted earlier, only F1, F2, and F3 (the first three peaks starting from the left) are of particular interest. As can be seen for /w/, F1 and F2 are very close together with a large gap between F2 and F3. Contrast this with a normal /r/ in which the peak for F2 has moved up slightly in frequency. Also, the peak for F3 has dropped considerably in frequency making it much closer to F2. As discussed in the section Spectrogram Displays, this narrowing of the distance between F2 and F3 is the classic pattern that captures the nature of American English /r/. The bottom panel in Figure 10–2 represents a derhotacized /r/. Productions of a derhotacized /r/ can vary considerably from example to example and from speaker to speaker, and so the displays also vary considerably. Productions that are closer to /w/ will have the F3 peak shifted further to the right. In this case, F3 the production was closer to /r/, and the peak for F3 has moved closer to F2 but is much smaller.

BASICS OF VISUAL ACOUSTIC FEEDBACK[2]

As with tactile feedback and EPG, visual acoustic feedback is intended as a supplement to some overall therapy structure such as traditional articulation therapy, and it is intended to assist primarily with the

---

[2]Detailed instructions for any particular acoustic analysis system are beyond the scope of this book, as there are the many variations across systems and software packages. Developers of each system typically provide some level of instruction regarding their use. See also Neel (2010).

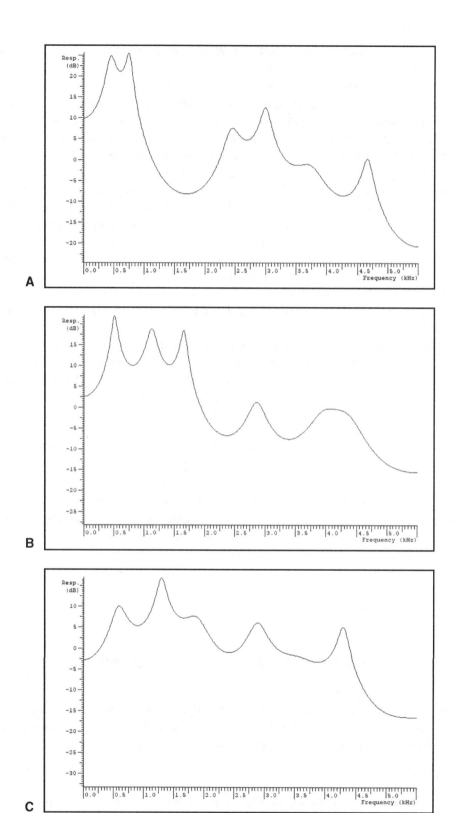

Figure 10–2. Examples of linear predictive coding spectra. **A.** Normal /w/. **B.** Normal /r/. **C.** Derhotacized /r/. Images generated by Dr. Amy Neel.

establishment phase of therapy. The basic idea is to allow the client to experiment with their articulators to match a target. This might be done while the clinician tries out a variety of elicitation techniques (Shuster et al., 1992).

Establishing a visual target depends on the circumstances and the particular acoustic software being used. First, because of age- and gender-related differences in formant frequencies, the target should be one that is ideally produced by someone matching the age and sex of the client. Once such a person is identified, recordings of the target sounds in isolation, syllables, and words can be made in advance. In cases where no matching target speaker is available, recordings can be made of each of the client's attempts, and the best attempts can be saved for use as the target. As the client's productions improve, the "target" sample can potentially change.

For spectrogram displays, if the software allows for split-screen presentation, the target can be displayed on one half of the screen, and the client's attempts can then be each displayed on the other half. With some programs that provide LPC displays (e.g., PENTAX Medical Sona-Match), the target version can be used as a template, and the client's production is actively overlaid on the template (i.e., both the target and what the client produces are visible simultaneously). As LPC displays represent dynamic real-time displays, the client can simply experiment live to try to get the formant peaks to line up with the template.

In cases where no split-screen is possible, a spectrogram target can be printed out and used to compare to the client's production. Where no overlay option is available for LPC displays, the target spectrum can be traced on a clear sheet of plastic, and this can be physically attached to the computer screen to serve as a template to be matched.

Orientation to Visual Acoustic Feedback

As with all new kinds of feedback, and in particular given the abstract nature of the images in visual acoustic feedback, orientation to the use of this technology will be necessary. Such orientation would occur following a baseline probe that would be recorded to serve as the basis for monitoring progress and generalization. This might involve conducting a stimulability probe as shown in Appendix 4–1 and measuring accuracy in conversation using the form in Appendix 4–3. The word-level probe found in Table 4–1 can also be administered. The particular words in that probe would then need to be excluded from therapy sessions.

Both McAllister Byun and Hitchcock (2012) and Hitchcock and Cabbage (2019) have suggested using the first two treatment sessions for such an orientation. An adaptation of their orientation processes is outlined in Table 10–1.

Table 10–1. Possible Orientation Plan for Use With Visual Acoustic Feedback

Session 1	Introduce the system
	Demonstrate output with /i/ and /u/
	Orient client to the image on the screen
	Display recorded vowel examples and have client guess which they are
	Demonstrate /r/
	Orient them to the low distance between F2 and F3
	Check client comprehension
Session 2	Introduce idea of model (template) matching
	Have client try to match vowel models
	Try elicitation techniques to obtain a good /r/
	Introduce models (if available) or record best production
	Have client try to match model with different elicitation techniques
	Check client comprehension

Note. Adapted from *Biofeedback for Childhood Speech Disorders: Practical Information for Clinicians* [Webinar], by E. R. Hitchcock and K. Cabbage, November 2019, presented to American Speech-Language-Hearing Association Special Interest Groups 1, 16, and 19; and "Investigating the Use of Traditional and Spectral Feedback for Approaches to Intervention for /r/ Misarticulation," by T. McAllister Byun and E. R. Hitchcock, 2012, *American Journal of Speech-Language Pathology*, 21, 207–221 (https://doi.org/10.1044/1058-0360(2012/11-0083).

Establishment and Stabilization With
Visual Acoustic Feedback

Following orientation, the initial goal is to try to get the client to consistently produce a correct /r/. The intent is to get them to do whatever they need to do to match the visual acoustic model provided. One approach might be to simply tell them to experiment with their tongue after the target sound is modeled for them. As an example, the client in the case study by Shuster and colleagues (1992) "was instructed to produce an [ɝ] and then to move his tongue around to 'move the formants around'" (p. 32). We might also provide some phonetic placement instruction (i.e., describe what they might do). If that proved unsuccessful as it did for the participant in the Shuster et al. (1992) study, various elicitation techniques could be combined with the visual acoustic feedback. For example, Shuster et al. (1992) elicited /r/ using a combination of shaping from /l/ (see Shriberg, 1975; also outlined in Appendix 6–1) and spectrogram feedback. Another option would be to explore different facilitating contexts. For example, in the study by Shuster, Ruscello, and Toth (1995), their female participant was more successful using front vowel contexts (e.g., /ir/), while their male participant was more successful using back vowel contexts (e.g., /or/).

Once correct production is obtained, the client would be asked to repeat this multiple times to reinforce the movement and placement. Feedback from the visual acoustic display and the clinician's perceptual judgments about correctness would be the reinforcement. Whenever an incorrect production was noted, the elicitation technique that had worked to help them reach a correct /r/ might be reintroduced as a reminder cue to help them get back to correct production.

Moving from establishment to stabilization will require fading out the visual acoustic feedback. This may begin at the isolation, syllable, or word level. As discussed in Chapter 9 for EPG, one approach might be to systematically fade it out within each session. For example, over the course of a session, the visual acoustic feedback could be reduced from 100% of trials (every trial) to 50% (every other trial) to 0% (no use) to encourage generalization to production without the feedback. At subsequent sessions, the visual acoustic feedback would be available if needed.

As discussed previously, the generalization phase would begin once some preset level was reached. Although there is no solid evidence suggesting what that ideal point might be, one possibility is to use success at the real-word level (e.g., 80% correct or higher) without the feedback. From this point onward, the visual acoustic feedback (and/or the elicitation technique that was used to obtain a correct /r/) would again be available to provide reminders if production accuracy became too low at higher levels in the treatment hierarchy.

EVIDENCE FOR VISUAL ACOUSTIC FEEDBACK WITH /r/ ERRORS

Several published studies have provided evidence for the efficacy of visual acoustic feedback for remediating /r/ errors. These are highlighted chronologically in Table 10–2.

In all five studies, the findings indicated improvement in /r/ accuracy with visual acoustic feedback for the majority of the participants using the feedback and some amount of generalization to untreated targets without the feedback. This suggests that visual acoustic feedback can be effective at remediating /r/ errors. However, it does not work in all cases. It is not clear whether this lack of universal success reflects the difficulty in breaking highly ingrained bad habits or the challenge that some clients might have with relating to the abstract feedback being provided. More study might help sort this out.

Table 10–2. Summary of Available Evidence for Use of Visual Acoustic Feedback to Remediate /r/

Study (evidence level)	Population	Sample	Design	Feedback Method	Tx Schedule	Outcomes
Shuster et al., 1992 (Level III)	18-year-old	$n = 1$ male	AB design	Spectrograms	Three Tx sessions (50 min)	0% accuracy after 17 traditional Tx sessions. 100% correct in isolation for three sessions following withdrawal of visual acoustic feedback.
Shuster et al., 1995 (Level IIb)	Older children 0% accuracy after 2 to 4 years of traditional Tx	$n = 2$ 10-year-old male 14-year-old female	AB design repeated across participants	Spectrograms	Male: two times per week (50 min) Female: one time per week (1 hr)	Male: 83%+ correct in words without acoustic feedback after 24 Tx sessions. Continued progress with traditional Tx and dismissed the next semester. Female: 100% correct /r/ in words without visual acoustic feedback after 10 Tx sessions. Generalization reported to conversation in traditional Tx sessions.

Study (evidence level)	Population	Sample	Design	Feedback Method	Tx Schedule	Outcomes
McAllister Byun and Hitchcock, 2012 (Level Ib)	6;0 to 11;9 Most had 1 to 4 years of traditional Tx with little or no success on /r/	$n = 11$ (10 males, 1 female)	Multiple baselines across participants (with random assignment)	LPC displays	Two times per week (30 min) for 10 weeks 4 to 6 weeks of traditional Tx then 4 to 6 weeks of visual acoustic Tx	9 of 11 participants showed no change prior to visual acoustic feedback. 8 of 11 made some within-session improvement with visual acoustic feedback. 4 of 11 showed generalization to untreated words.
McAllister Byun et al., 2016 (Level IIa)	6;8 to 13;3 At least 5 months of prior Tx for /r/ without success	$n = 9$ (6 males, 3 females)	Multiple baselines across participants and behaviors (different variants of /r/)	LPC displays with or without articulatory cues (internal versus external focus)	Two times per week (30 min) for 8 weeks	6 of 9 participants showed improvement on at least one variant of /r/. No advantage for internal or external focus of attention.
McAllister Byun and Campbell, 2016 (Level Ib)	9;3 to 15;10 Most had some prior Tx for /r/ All initially less than 25% correct in words	$n = 11$ (7 males, 4 females)	Multiple baselines across participants (with random assignment) Also crossover design; visual acoustic versus traditional Tx	LPC displays	All received both Tx types Randomly assigned to either acoustic feedback or traditional Tx first 20 total Tx sessions	7/11 participants showed meaningful improvement overall. 4/11 participants showed no meaningful response to either Tx. Similar effect sizes for both Tx types. Larger effect sizes for visual acoustic feedback when administered first.

Note. Tx = treatment.

SPECIFIC EQUIPMENT FOR VISUAL ACOUSTIC FEEDBACK

A variety of different systems are available for providing visual acoustic feedback. They vary in their complexity, cost, and amount of support being provided. Although all system developers provide some level of instruction and support for their systems, not surprisingly, it is generally true that the less the systems cost, the less clinician friendly the support will be.

Starting with the most expensive and most advanced systems, PENTAX Medical offers several commercial products that can be used to provide visual acoustic feedback. They include systems with proprietary hardware such as their research quality Computerized Speech Lab (CSL) system, and their Visi-Pitch system, which is an advanced clinical program. They also offer their Sona-Speech II system that is a clinical software program that runs on a laptop computer Details about these products can be found online (https://www.pentaxmedical.com/pentax/service/usa).

An Australian company called Multimedia Speech Pathology offers a variety of commercial clinical tools including a visual acoustic feedback program called TheraVox (more details at https://mmsp.com.au/product/theravox-voice-and-speech-biofeedback-activities/).

There is also a range of free programs available. Two fairly comprehensive programs include Praat (which is the Dutch word for "talk"; downloadable from http://www.fon.hum.uva.nl/praat/) and wavesurfer.js (downloadable at https://wavesurfer-js.org/). Both of these are capable of multiple analyses but will require some time investment to learn how to use them. However, the developers provide some basic tutorials. An online search will also lead to several tutorials developed by others.

Several other free programs that each provide specific kinds of feedback were developed by Professor Mark Huckvale at University College, London. These include WASP, which provides waveform, spectrogram, and fundamental frequency displays, and RTSpect, which provides real-time spectrum displays. Details on downloading these and some other related programs can be found on the Internet (https://www.speechandhearing.net/).

Finally, a free iPad app called staRt (speech therapist's app for /R/ treatment) has been developed by Dr. Tara McAllister and her colleagues at New York University. It was specifically intended for clinicians working on remediation of /r/ and provides LPC display feedback. It can be downloaded at the iOS App Store (more details at https://wp.nyu.edu/byunlab/projects/start/).

SUMMARY

Visual acoustic feedback has been shown to be effective for some clients with /r/ errors. It offers several advantages including (a) available free software, (b) real-time feedback, and (c) use not limited to any particular tongue shape. One notable disadvantage of this type of feedback is that some clients may have difficulty relating to the abstract nature of the images.

In the next chapter, our attention turns to our last treatment option and the most recently developed visual feedback option, ultrasound.

CHAPTER 11[1]

Treatment Option 6: Adding Visual Feedback via Ultrasound

In this final treatment-specific chapter, the focus is on ultrasound, which is also the most recently developed visual feedback option. This approach uses the same technology now regularly used for prenatal examinations and many other medical imaging procedures. Although it has apparently been used in some form since as far back as the 1940s, the first commercially available ultrasound systems were not produced until the 1960s.

Ultrasound involves using high-frequency sound waves (above the range of normal human hearing) directed toward the intended image site. Variations in the amount of sound being reflected back are converted to an image by specific software. Multiple images are being created per second, allowing it to be useful for monitoring fast-moving speech movements. A few early studies of this tool and speech were conducted in the 1980s (e.g., Shawker & Sonies, 1985), with most research and clinical reports appearing in the last 15 to 20 years. In addition to its use with individuals with persistent and residual /r/ errors, it has been used with other speech sound targets (e.g., Cleland et al., 2019). Ultrasound has also shown some efficacy for speech remediation with other populations including individuals with hearing impairment (e.g., Bacsfalvi, 2010; Bacsfalvi & Bernhardt, 2011), those with childhood apraxia of speech (e.g., Preston et al.,

---

[1]If you have not already done so, it might be useful to review the general information on feedback in the first few pages of Chapter 8 and information on visual feedback in particular in the first few pages of Chapter 9.

2013, 2016), learners of English as a second language (e.g., Gick et al., 2008), adults with Down syndrome (e.g., Fawcett et al., 2008), and those who have undergone partial glossectomy (e.g., Blythe et al., 2016).

Ultrasound offers at least four advantages for speech remediation. First, it can give a direct view of all parts of the vocal tract including the pharynx simultaneously. As such, it eliminates all the guesswork about tongue placement and movement. For remediation of /r/, such a perspective is valuable because it can provide a simultaneous view of both internal constrictions (i.e., at the palate and in the pharynx), allowing the client to manipulate both at the same time. Second, by simply rotating the probe head 90 degrees, a front-to-back view of the vocal tract can be changed to a left-to-right view, or vice versa. This effectively means being able to see all aspects of tongue configuration (i.e., both specific constriction locations and any tongue-to-palate contact). The third advantage of ultrasound is that, like electropalatography (EPG) and visual acoustic (linear predictive coding) feedback, the information is being conveyed to the client in real time. Finally, unlike some other options that have been discussed, it is not limited to any particular tongue shape. The client can literally experiment with any combination of tongue movements and constrictions while observing both the vocal tract shape that results and listening for the sound that is produced. The one major disadvantage of ultrasound remains its cost. Although portable ultrasound systems have become significantly less expensive in recent years, most clinicians are unlikely to be able to spend the several thousand dollars required. The use of ultrasound is discussed here because of its great remediation potential and the fact that it is starting to be used in some large hospitals and other private practice situations. A possible consultative model for its use in other settings is discussed later.

For the sake of completeness and in case the reader has not reviewed the earlier chapters, a few important reminders are in order at this point. First, it is assumed that, if used, ultrasound feedback by itself is not sufficient for successful speech sound remediation. The assumption is that it will be used as part of some systematic therapy structure such as traditional articulation therapy. Second, as with other alternative forms of feedback, its use is intended primarily as part of the establishment phase of therapy. Third, as suggested by Hitchcock and Cabbage (2019), ideal candidates for therapy involving any supplemental visual input should have normal vision, have normal cognitive skills (i.e., be able to understand the images), and be able to sit and attend well. This would typically mean that ultrasound feedback is likely best suited for children who are 7 years old and older. The fact that it has been used successfully with individuals with Down syndrome suggests that it should not be immediately ruled out with those who have cognitive impairments or with younger children.

ULTRASOUND AS A TYPE OF FEEDBACK

In general, ultrasound feedback provides the client with information about what the articulators are doing. In this case, the client and the clinician can both see in real time what is happening in all parts of the vocal tract, including the pharynx. In Chapter 5, in the discussion of principles of motor learning, knowing what the articulators are doing was referred to as knowledge of performance (KP) feedback. While receiving such feedback, the client may also be receiving feedback from the clinician about whether or not the target sound was produced correctly (knowledge of results or KR feedback). The evidence discussed in Chapter 5 suggested that over time, KP feedback should be changed to KR feedback. Making this change allows the client to become their own therapist by combining the KR feedback with the feedback they receive from their own articulators and what they hear. Thus, to be consistent with principles of motor learning, ultrasound feedback must be faded out over time to allow this switch to take place.

Box 11–1

Reminder: Ultrasound feedback is intended largely for the establishment phase of therapy.

As therapy progresses to stabilization and generalization, the new feedback must be faded out.

BASICS OF ULTRASOUND FEEDBACK

Ultrasound technology uses sound waves at frequencies between 1 and 20 MHz, which are well above the range of normal human hearing (which does not extend much past 20 kHz). Each ultrasound system uses specific frequencies; some provide frequency options, while others are limited to a single frequency. According to Lee, Wrench, and Sancibrian (2015), tongue movements are most often examined using the frequency range of 2 to 7.5 MHz. Systems can include multiple hardware components, but the simplest ones include only a probe (also called a transducer) connected to a personal computer with ultrasound software installed. Differences between simpler and more advanced systems apparently represent mostly the range of different functions available, not image quality. Lee et al. suggest that most advanced ultrasound functions are not used in speech remediation. For example, Cleland, Scobbie, and Wrench (2015) note that systems vary in terms of the rate of image capture that is measured in number of frames per second (fps). A rate of 18 fps "is adequate for viewing dynamic movements during therapy" (p. 576), but rates of 60 to 200 fps would be needed if simultaneous acoustic analysis were also required. Put another way, the simpler and less expensive systems may be sufficient for most speech remediation applications. It is not, however, just a matter of selecting a simpler system. Ultrasound systems are often not designed only for speech therapy applications and thus may vary considerably in terms of features and specifications across manufacturers and models. The reader is referred to Lee et al. (2015) and Stone (2005) for some guidance on the technical aspects of selecting specific ultrasound systems for speech remediation purposes.

Regardless of the system being used, the ultrasound probe is positioned under the client's chin as shown in Figure 11–1. Prior to positioning, ultrasound gel is applied to the skin to ensure complete contact and to prevent any air gaps that would interfere with both sending and receiving the ultrasound signal.

The probe is typically held in one position (i.e., is not moved around), but it can be oriented two different ways depending on the desired view. Orienting it along the midsagittal plane provides a view of the vocal tract from front to back and allows for viewing of the overall tongue shape and the constrictions being created. Turning the probe 90 degrees and orienting it along the coronal plane provides a left-to-right view of the oral cavity. For tongue imaging, this allows the clinician and client to see whether

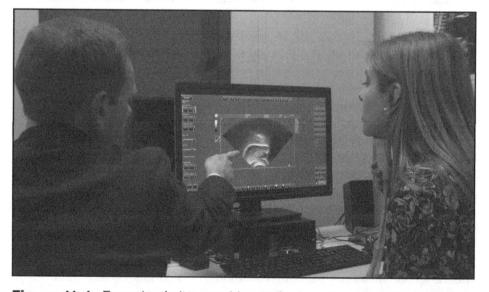

Figure 11–1. Example of ultrasound in use for speech remediation. Copyright 2020 Jonathan L. Preston. Reprinted with permission. All Rights Reserved.

the sides of the tongue body are up and contacting the upper teeth (as expected for a tongue tip down or bunched tongue shape). It also allows for a view of the center of the tongue which should be forming a groove for air and sound to travel through. The coronal view does not provide any view of the back of the tongue. Examples of midsagittal and coronal views are shown in Figure 11–2.

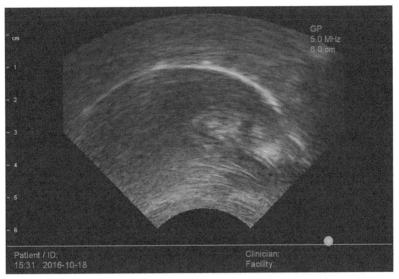

A

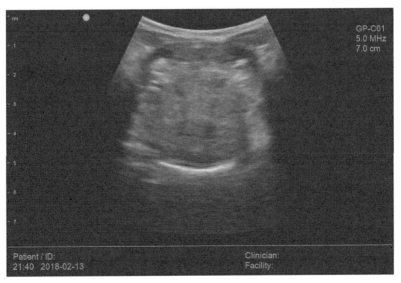

B

Figure 11–2. Sagittal (**A**) and coronal (**B**) ultrasound views of the adult tongue. Copyright 2020 SeeMore Imaging Canada. Reprinted with permission. All Rights Reserved.

For purposes of tracking progress, it is always useful to make recordings. Lee et al. (2015) note that while most ultrasound systems allow for image recording, most are not set up to simultaneously record sound. Given that multiple tongue shapes may be used to achieve a perceptually acceptable /r/, such recordings would be crucial to understanding how successful the client is being at reaching the target. Lee et al. recommend the use of screen capture software such as CamStudio to make such recordings.

Clinician Training and Orientation

Unlike most of the other options being discussed in this book, clinicians who wish to make use of ultrasound for speech remediation will need to become familiar with its use. This includes understanding the operation and maintenance of the specific equipment as well as optimizing and (perhaps more importantly) understanding the images that are being displayed. Given variations in equipment and possible settings, detailed instruction is beyond the scope of this book. Readers are referred to published studies for some additional background. A clinician resource manual developed by Cleland and colleagues (2018) may also be quite helpful in this regard. It offers a series of examples, including videos, of using ultrasound for speech remediation (available from https://doi .org/10.15129/63372). Note that the manual is not focused exclusively on remediation of /r/ though it includes some discussion of it. It should also be noted that the manual was developed around a particular ultrasound system though much of the information being presented is generic enough for application to other systems.

Overcoming Cost Concerns

The cost of ultrasound equipment has declined considerably in the last 10 years, but it can still cost thousands of dollars even for a fairly simple system. This would normally make it out of reach for many clinicians. However, alternative service delivery models may offer a potential for providing access to this treatment option. A 2008 Canadian study by Bernhardt and colleagues, for example, demonstrated how a consultative model with ultrasound might work for clients in rural areas without access to expensive technology. Local speech-language pathologists (SLPs) provided initial traditional treatment with little or no success. This was followed by a short series of ultrasound sessions conducted by SLPs trained in ultrasound use who traveled to the rural communities. The visits included a short workshop for the local SLP on the goals and procedures involved with ultrasound. During the consultation visit, each client was trained to establish a correct /r/ using ultrasound, and the local clinician subsequently worked with the client through the stabilization and generalization phases using traditional therapy. Of the 13 school-age participants in the Bernhardt et al. study, 11 showed improvement in /r/ accuracy after receiving ultrasound treatment. The four children who participated in more and longer ultrasound sessions made the greatest gains. Such a model might be replicated across a school district or health authority where one system was purchased and one to two clinicians were trained to provide the consultative service.

Addressing Safety Concerns

Ultrasound imaging is generally regarded as safe as it does not involve the use of ionizing radiation. However, according to Lee, Wrench, and Sancibrian (2015), caution should be exercised as "it is a form of energy which, above certain thresholds, can cause tissue heating and/or interaction effects with microscopic bubbles in the body" (p. 72). This may be a particular concern for speech remediation as the duration of ultrasound exposure is typically longer than for most other imaging applications. Lee et al. offer several suggestions for minimizing exposure including (a) selecting a probe frequency only as high as necessary to get the desired image (higher frequencies require more power); (b) setting output power as low as possible, while using the gain setting to compensate for lower power settings; (c) freezing the display (which stops the sound generation) when not using the feedback; and (d) making sure the probe is turned off when not in contact with the skin.

To mitigate any infection risks, the ultrasound probe should be cleaned and disinfected following each use.

Orientation to Ultrasound Feedback

Similar to any new technology, ultrasound will require some amount of orientation so that the client can become familiar with the equipment being used and the feedback being provided. Such orientation would take place following a baseline probe that would be recorded to serve as the basis for monitoring progress and generalization. Such a probe might involve testing stimulability as shown in Appendix 4–1 and measuring production accuracy in conversation using the form in Appendix 4–3. The word-level probe found in Table 4–1 could also be administered. The particular words in that probe would then need to be excluded from therapy sessions.

Several sources have discussed the need for ultrasound orientation (Bernhardt et al., 2008; Cleland et al., 2015; Hitchcock & Cabbage, 2019). Considering all of their suggestions, a possible ultrasound orientation outline is shown in Table 11–1.

Table 11–1. Possible Orientation Plan for Use With Ultrasound Feedback

Session 1	Introduce the system
	Review anatomy
	Orient client to the image on the screen with midsagittal view
	Discuss different tongue shapes for /r/
	Demonstrate different tongue shapes with clinician models
	Have client try to reproduce different tongue shapes without any sound
	Try phonetic placement cues to elicit correct /r/
	Check client comprehension
Session 2	Introduce coronal view
	Have client try to reproduce different tongue shapes without any sound
	Try phonetic placement cues to elicit correct /r/
	Check client comprehension

Note. Adapted from Bernhardt et al. (2008), Cleland et al. (2015), and Hitchcock & Cabbage (2019). "Ultrasound as Visual Feedback in Speech Habilitation: Exploring Consultative Use in Rural British Columbia," by B. M. Bernhardt, P. Bacsfalvi, M. Adler-Bock, R. Shimizu, A. Cheney, N. Giesbrecht, M. O'Connell, J. Sirianni, and B. Radanov, 2008, *Clinical Linguistics and Phonetics*, *22*(2), 149–162 (https://doi .org/10.1080/02699200701801225); "Using Ultrasound Visual Feedback to Treat Persistent Primary Speech Sound Disorders," by J. Cleland, J. M. Scobbie, and A. A. Wrench, 2015, *Clinical Linguistics and Phonetics*, *29*(8–10), 575–597 (https:// doi.org/10.3109/02699206.2015.1016188); and *Biofeedback for Childhood Speech Disorders: Practical Information for Clinicians* [Webinar], by E. R. Hitchcock and K. Cabbage, November 2019, presented to American Speech-Language-Hearing Association Special Interest Groups 1, 16, and 19.

Two comments are appropriate here. First, clinician models could include either prerecorded samples or having the clinician demonstrate in front of the child so they can also see how the process works. Second, the goal of client attempts to produce different tongue shapes without sound is to focus their attention specifically on the movements and the resulting change in the visual feedback. Removing the auditory output may be especially helpful for some therapy-resistant clients.

Establishment and Stabilization With Ultrasound Feedback

As with all other approaches, the initial goal is to establish correct target production. Doing so may require some experimentation given that to date no particular tongue shape for /r/ has proven to be universally successful. McAllister Byun et al. (2014) suggest that the client be given opportunities to explore different tongue shapes. Such exploration need not be random but can be guided by systematic use of a variety of elicitation techniques. Similar to the discussion of EPG, once a good production is generated, a clear plastic sheet can be placed on the computer screen, and the tongue shape can be traced. This can serve as the target tongue shape model for the client. The resulting ultrasound images can also be saved for future reference. As with all other approaches, the tongue shape target need not be completely fixed. If the client fails to progress, other tongue shapes can be attempted.

Relative to the stabilization phase, a possible treatment sequence adapted from Cleland et al. (2018) is shown in Table 11–2.

Cleland et al. (2018) suggest a progress criterion of 80% correct for moving to next steps. Note in Table 11–2 that fading out of the ultrasound feedback begins fairly early in the sequence (Step 4) to ensure generalization to production without the ultrasound.

Table 11–2. Suggested Treatment Sequence for /r/ Stabilization With Ultrasound

Step	Target
1	/r/ + facilitative vowel (as CV or VC depending on what works best)
2	/r/ + V with a variety of vowels
3	V + /r/ with a variety of vowels
4	/r/ + VC sequences[a]
5	CV + /r/ sequences
6	Multisyllabic words[b]
7	Imitated phrases with /r/ initial words
8	Imitated phrases with /r/ final words
9	Sentence completion tasks with variety of /r/ target words
10	Words containing /r/ clusters
11	Imitated sentences with a variety of /r/ words
12	Spontaneous sentences with a variety of /r/ words

Note. Adapted from *ULTRAX2020: Ultrasound Technology for Optimising the Treatment of Speech Disorders* [Clinicians' Resource Manual], by J. Cleland, A. Wrench, S. Lloyd, and E. Sugden, 2018 (https://doi.org/10.15129/63372).

[a]Begin fading out ultrasound feedback.

[b]Increasingly fade out ultrasound feedback.

Once ultrasound feedback has been faded out, the generalization phase would begin. From this point onward, the elicitation technique that was used to obtain a correct /r/ (or perhaps ultrasound feedback if still available) would only be used on occasion to provide reminders if production accuracy became too low at higher levels in the treatment hierarchy.

EVIDENCE FOR ULTRASOUND FEEDBACK FOR /r/ ERRORS

Despite the relative newness of ultrasound feedback for speech remediation, there appear to be more studies of its efficacy than most of the other alternative approaches presented in this book. A systematic review by Sugden, Lloyd, Lam, and Cleland (2019) identified 29 empirical studies with most having been published in the last 15 years. Most used single-subject designs and included from 1 to 13 participants varying in age from 4 to 27 years (mean age of 11 years). Of the 103 unique individuals studied, most (83) were treated for /r/ errors. Sugden and colleagues concluded that ultrasound (a) can help establish production of speech targets but does not, by itself, facilitate generalization; (b) can be used successfully with a variety of speech sound targets and appears to be especially useful for /r/; and (c) can be an effective supplement to more traditional therapy. They noted, however, that similar to the bulk of the research in speech sound disorders, much of the evidence is lower level (Level IIb or III) and includes small samples. Additional study is clearly needed. The recent noticeable increase in the number of studies being published is a clear, positive sign.

As with the other approaches discussed in this book, ultrasound feedback does not appear to be universally successful for speech remediation. Sugden et al. (2019) noted that 10 of the 29 studies (35%) reported mixed findings, where some participants either failed to respond overall or showed poor generalization to untreated items. It is not yet possible to identify specific participant or treatment characteristics that might affect treatment outcomes.

SPECIFIC ULTRASOUND EQUIPMENT

Studies of speech remediation with ultrasound have used several different specific devices (see Lee et al., 2015, for a discussion). Many of the devices included in the published literature have been discontinued, although at least two viable systems are currently available.

A Canadian company called SeeMore Imaging markets two different models specifically intended for speech-language pathology application. Both are probes intended to connect to PC-based laptop computers (details found at https://seemore.ca/portable-ultrasound-products/).

The British company Articulate Instruments markets a system specifically for speech-language pathology application. It includes a probe and some additional hardware. Matching software is available that allows for synchronized audio recording for acoustic analysis. More information can be found on the Internet (http://www.articulateinstruments.com/ultrasound-imaging/?target=Echo%20B).

SUMMARY

Available evidence suggests that ultrasound can assist some individuals with establishment of /r/ when used in conjunction with motor-based treatment such as traditional articulation therapy. It offers at least four advantages for speech remediation. First, it offers a direct view of all parts of the vocal tract including the pharynx, thus eliminating all the guesswork about tongue placement and movement. For remediation of /r/, in particular, it can provide a simultaneous view of both internal constrictions (i.e., at the palate and in the pharynx), allowing the client to manipulate both at the same time. Second, it offers both a front-to-back view and a left-to-right view for examining both specific constriction locations and any tongue-to-teeth contact. Third, the information is being conveyed to the client in real time. Finally, it is not limited to any particular tongue shape. The major disadvantage of ultrasound remains its cost.

CHAPTER 12

Concluding Remarks: Deciding What to Do

Given the available menu of options, how does one decide which approach to use? Although there are few direct comparisons across approaches (some are underway as of this writing), a first step might be to compare the relative advantages and disadvantages of each option. A summary is presented in Table 12–1.

One thing that is clear is that none of the available options stands out as the obvious choice. Short of that, clinicians must consider their own situation. In so doing, there are clearly several factors to consider.

Cost is clearly an issue for most clinicians working in the public schools. Budgets have long been tight and are likely to remain so for the foreseeable future. That said, three of the seven options discussed (fine-tuning traditional therapy, concurrent treatment, visual acoustic feedback) are essentially free. Of the remainder, Systematic Articulation Training Program Accessing Computers (SATPAC) and Speech Buddies only require a modest investment that some parents or school districts may be able to manage. The cost of electropalatography (EPG) has come down considerably in recent years but remains largely out of reach for those working in the schools. On the other hand, the recent reductions in cost likely explain why EPG is fast becoming a viable option in many private practice situations. Finally, ultrasound, the newest option and the one that offers the most complete view of the articulation of /r/, is currently the least accessible for most clinicians simply because of the costs involved. In situations where multiple clinicians work for the same employer, consideration might be given to making the cost more manageable by using a consultation approach, which was discussed in Chapter 11.

Table 12–1. Summary of the Advantages and Disadvantages of Available[a] Options for Remediating /r/

Option	Chapter	Advantages	Disadvantages
Fine-tuning traditional articulation therapy	6	Free Not limited to any particular tongue shape	May not be motivating enough for some therapy-resistant clients.
Concurrent treatment	7	Free Not limited to any particular tongue shape	Random order may be disconcerting for some clinicians or confusing for some clients.
SATPAC	7	Extensive use of nonwords may be key to breaking bad habits for some clients Not limited to any particular tongue shape	Cost $.
Speech Buddies	8	Consistent placement and tactile feedback in real time Device can be used at home by parents	Cost $. Can only target retroflex /r/. Possible client aversion to foreign objects in the mouth.
EPG	9	Somewhat direct view of what the tongue is doing in real time Real-time feedback	Cost $$. Can only target bunched /r/. Possible client aversion to foreign objects in the mouth. Pseudopalate may no longer fit well if teeth change.
Visual acoustic feedback	10	Free software available Real-time feedback Not limited to any particular tongue shape	Abstract images may be difficult for some clients to relate to.
Ultrasound	11	Direct view of all areas of the vocal tract Real-time feedback Not limited to any particular tongue shape	Cost $$$.

Note. EPG = electropalatography; SATPAC = Systematic Articulation Training Program Accessing Computers.

[a]Only approaches that would be available to most clinicians and that appear to be appropriate for children with persistent and residual speech errors (i.e., usually only one to two errors) were included.

For therapy-resistant clients with long-established bad habits, adopting a very different approach to shake things up a bit might be worth considering to get past the resistance. All of the approaches presented (except possibly fine tuning of traditional therapy) offer the potential to do that. They either involve radically modifying traditional treatment (concurrent treatment, SATPAC), or they offer forms of alternative feedback (Speech Buddies, visual acoustic feedback, EPG, ultrasound) that may motivate some clients to work more diligently toward their therapy goals.

The fact that none of the approaches discussed are universally successful highlights a long-standing problem with speech sound disorders that was discussed in some detail in Chapter 5. This has been highlighted by Farquharson (2019) and was mentioned by Cleland et al. (2019), among others. Treatment should focus on the actual problem, and all of the approaches discussed in this book share one basic assumption. They start with the premise that the problem with single sound errors is motor based (i.e., that it is an articulation disorder). Clinicians need to consider the very real possibility that some of these clients have either perceptual or phonological problems underlying their speech errors, either as an alternative diagnosis or in addition to motor issues. In such cases, nonmotor approaches may be more appropriate or need to be applied concurrently. Some suggestions for assessment of these other potential problems are provided in Chapter 4 with treatment options discussed in Chapter 5.

This brings an end to the tour of possible treatment options for remediating /r/ errors. Three closing comments should be made at this point. First, to recall a point made at the outset of our journey, although the focus has primarily been on older children with persistent and residual errors, the approaches discussed could certainly be applied to other populations. (The visual feedback options, especially acoustics and EPG, are likely limited to those over 7 years of age.) Second, while the empirical evidence for each of the approaches that were discussed is limited, what is available suggests that each approach appears to be helpful for at least some individuals. Finally, while this represents the range of options that is currently available, given the challenges of /r/, there is every reason to believe that researchers and clinicians alike will continue to be motivated to develop additional options. However, we need not wait. The bottom line, and the reason why this book was written, is that viable options exist now.

References

Adams, S. G., & Page, A. D. (2000). Effects of selected practice and feedback variables on speech motor learning. *Journal of Medical Speech-Language Pathology, 8*(4), 215–220.

American Speech-Language-Hearing Association. (2005). *Evidence-based practice in communication disorders* [Position statement]. https://doi.org/10.1044/policy.PS2005-00221

Arlt, P. B., & Goodban, M. T. (1976). A comparative study of articulation acquisition as based on a study of 240 normals, aged three to six. *Language, Speech, and Hearing Services in Schools, 7*, 173–180. https://doi.org/10.1044/0161-1461.0703.173

Arndt, W., Elbert, M., & Shelton, R. (1970). Standardization of a test of oral stereognosis. In J. F. Bosma (Ed.), *Second Symposium on Oral Sensation and Perception* (pp. 363–378). Charles Thomas.

Bacsfalvi, P. (2010). Attaining the lingual components of /r/ with ultrasound for three adolescents with cochlear implants. *Canadian Journal of Speech-Language Pathology and Audiology, 34*(3), 206–217. https://cjslpa.ca/files/2010_CJSLPA_Vol_34/No_03_153-225/Bacsfalvi_CJSLPA_2010.pdf

Bacsfalvi, P., & Bernhardt, B. M. (2011). Long-term outcomes of speech therapy for seven adolescents with visual feedback technologies: Ultrasound and electropalatography. *Clinical Linguistics and Phonetics, 25*(11–12), 1034–1043. https://doi.org/10.3109/02699206.2011.618236

Bankson, N. W., & Bernthal, J. E. (1990). *Bankson-Bernthal test of phonology.* Pro-Ed.

Bankson, N. W., & Bernthal, J. E. (2019). *Bankson-Bernthal test of phonology* (2nd ed.). Pro-Ed.

Bernhardt, B. M., Bacsfalvi, P., Adler-Bock, M., Shimizu, R., Cheney, A. Giesbrecht, N., O'Connell, M., Sirianni, J., & Radanov, B. (2008). Ultrasound as visual feedback in speech habilitation: Exploring consultative use in rural British Columbia. *Clinical Linguistics and Phonetics, 22*(2), 149–162. https://doi.org/10.1080/02699200701801225

Bernthal, J. E., Bankson, N. W., & Flipsen, P., Jr. (2017). *Articulation and phonological disorders: Speech sound disorders in children* (8th ed.). Pearson Education.

Bleile, K. M. (2018). *The late eight* (3rd ed.). Plural Publishing.

Blythe, K. M., Mccabe, P., Madill, C., & Ballard, K. J. (2016). Ultrasound visual feedback in articulation therapy following partial glossectomy. *Journal of Communication Disorders, 61*, 1–15. https://doi.org/10.1016/j.jcomdis.2016.02.004

Borshart, C. (2016). *The easy R therapy program*. Speech Dynamics.

Bowers, L., & Huisingh, R. (2010). *LinguiSystems articulation test*. LinguiSystems.

Boyce, S. E. (2015). The articulatory phonetics of /r/ for residual speech errors. *Seminars in Speech and Language, 36*, 257–270. https://doi.org/10.1055/s-0035-1562909

Boyce, S., & Espy-Wilson, C. Y. (1997). Coarticulatory stability in American English /r/. *Journal of the Acoustical Society of America, 101*(6), 3741–3753. https://doi.org/10.1121/1.418333

Boyce, S. E., Tiede, M., Espy-Wilson, C., & Groves-Wright, K. (2015, August). Diversity of tongue shapes for the American English rhotic liquid. *Proceedings of the International Congress of Phonetic Sciences*. International Phonetic Association.

Brumbaugh, K. M., & Smit, A. B. (2013). Treating children ages 3–6 who have speech sound disorder: A survey. *Language, Speech, and Hearing Services in Schools, 44*, 306–319. https://doi.org/10.1044/0161-1461(2013/12-0029)

Cabbage, K. L. (2015). The role of speech perception in persistent speech sound disorder. *Perspectives on School-Based Issues, 24*, 18–24. https://doi.org/10.1044/sbi16.2.18

Camarata, S. (2021). Naturalistic recast intervention. In A. L. Williams, S. McLeod, & R. J. McCauley (Eds.), *Interventions for speech sound disorders in children* (2nd ed., pp. 337–361). Paul H. Brookes Publishing.

Campbell, H., & McAllister Byun, T. (2018). Deriving individualised /r/ targets from the acoustics of children's non-rhotic vowels. *Clinical Linguistics and Phonetics, 32*(1), 70–87. https://doi.org/10.1080/02699206.2017.1330898

Carrier, J. K., Jr. (1970). A program of articulation therapy administered by mothers. *Journal of Speech and Hearing Disorders, 35*, 344–353. https://doi.org/10.1044/jshd.3504.344

Carter, P., & Edwards, S. (2004). EPG therapy for children with long-standing speech disorders: Predictions and outcomes. *Clinical Linguistics and Phonetics, 18*(6–8), 359–372. https://doi.org/10.1080/02699200410001703637

Christensen, M., & Hanson, M. (1981). An investigation of the efficacy of oral myofunctional therapy as a precursor to articulation therapy for pre–first grade children. *Journal of Speech and Hearing Disorders, 46*, 160–167. https://doi.org/10.1044/jshd.4602.160

Clark, C. E., Schwarz, I. E., & Blakeley, R. W. (1993). The removable R-appliance as a practice device to facilitate correct production of /r/. *American Journal of Speech-Language Pathology, 2*(1), 84–92. https://doi.org/10.1044/1058-0360.0201.84

Cleland, J., Scobbie, J. M., Roxburgh, Z., Heyde, C., & Wrench, A. (2019). Enabling new articulatory gestures in children with persistent and residual speech sound disorders using ultrasound visual biofeedback. *Journal of Speech, Language, and Hearing Research, 62*, 229 246. https://doi.org/10.1044/2018_JSLHR-S-17-0360

Cleland, J., Scobbie, J. M., & Wrench, A. A. (2015). Using ultrasound visual feedback to treat persistent primary speech sound disorders. *Clinical Linguistics and Phonetics, 29*(8–10), 575–597. https://doi.org/10.3109/02699 206.2015.1016188

Cleland, J., Timmins, C., Wood, S. E., Hardcastle, W. J., & Wishart, J. G. (2009). Electropalatographic therapy for children and young people with Down's syndrome. *Clinical Linguistics and Phonetics, 23*(12), 926–939. https://doi.org/10.3109/02699200903061776

Cleland, J., Wrench, A., Lloyd, S., & Sugden, E. (2018). *ULTRAX2020. Ultrasound technology for optimising the treatment of speech disorders* [Clinicians' resource manual]. https://doi.org/10.15129/63372

Cote, N. (2013, November). *Phonemic and tactile cueing for remediation of American English /r/: A case study* [Poster presentation]. Annual convention of the American Speech-Language-Hearing Association, Chicago, IL.

Cronin, S. A., Blanchet, P. G., Klonsky, B. B., & Piazza, N. (2014). The effect of a modeled /r/ articulatory disorder on listener perceptions of speech skills and personality traits. *Contemporary Issues in Communication Sciences and Disorders, 41*, 169–178. https://doi.org/10.1044/cicsd_41_F_169

Crowe, K., & McLeod, S. (2020). Children's English consonant acquisition in the United States: A review. *American Journal of Speech-Language Pathology, 29*, 2155–2169. https://doi.org/10.1044/2020_AJSLP-19-00168

Crowe Hall, B. J. (1991). Attitudes of fourth and sixth graders towards peers with mild articulation disorders. *Language, Speech, and Hearing Services in Schools, 22*, 334–340. https://doi.org/10.1044/0161-1461.2201.334

Curtis, J. F., & Hardy, J. C. (1959). A phonetic study of misarticulation of /r/. *Journal of Speech and Hearing Research, 2*(3), 244–257. https://doi.org/10.1044/jshr.0203.244

Dawson, J. I., & Tattersall, P. J. (2001). *Structured Photographic Articulation test-II featuring Dudsberry*. Janelle Publications.

Delattre, P., & Freeman, D. (1968). A dialect study of American r's by x-ray motion picture. *Linguistics, 44*, 29–68.

Dodd, B. J., Hua, Z., Crosbie, S., Holm, A., & Ozanne, A. (2006). *Diagnostic evaluation of articulation and phonology*. Pearson.

Duffy, J. R. (2005). *Motor speech disorders* (2nd ed.). Elsevier Mosby.

Dugan, S., Li, S. R., Masterson, J., Woeste, H., Mahalingam, N., Spencer, C., Mast, T. D., Riley, M. A., & Boyce, S. E. (2019). Tongue part movement trajectories for /r/ using ultrasound. *Perspectives of the ASHA Special Interest Groups, 4*, 1644–1652. https://doi.org/10.1044/2019_PERS-19-00064

Dworkin, J. P. (1978). A therapeutic technique for the improvement of lingua-alveolar valving abilities. *Language, Speech, and Hearing Services in Schools, 9*, 169–175. https://doi.org/10.1044/0161-1461.0903.169

Elbert, M., & McReynolds, L. V. (1975). Transfer of /r/ across contexts. *Journal of Speech and Hearing Disorders, 40*, 380–387. https://doi.org/10.1044/jshd.4003.380

Ertmer, D. J., & Maki, J. E. (2000). A comparison of speech training methods with deaf adolescents: Spectrographic versus noninstrumental instruction. *Journal of Speech, Language, and Hearing Research, 43*, 1509–1523. https://doi.org/10.1044/jslhr.4306.1509

Evans, C. M., & Potter, R. E. (1974). The effectiveness of the S-PACK when administered by sixth-grade children to primary grade children. *Language, Speech, and Hearing Services in Schools, 5*, 85–90. https://doi.org/10.1044/0161-1461.0502.85

Fabus, R., Raphael, L., Gatzonis, S., Dondorf, K., Giardina, K., Cron, S., & Badke, B. (2015). Preliminary case studies investigating the use of electropalatography (EPG) manufactured by CompleteSpeech® as a biofeedback tool in intervention. *International Journal of Linguistics and Communication, 3*(1), 11–23. https://doi.org/10.15640/ijlc.v3n1a3

Fant, G. (1973). *Speech sounds and features*. MIT Press.

Farquharson, K. (2019). It might not be "just artic": The case for the single sound error. *Perspectives of the ASHA Special Interest Groups, 4*, 76–84. https://doi.org/10.1044/2018_PERS-SIG1-2018-0019

Farquharson, K., & Boldini, L. (2018). Variability in interpreting "educational performance" for children with speech sound disorders. *Language, Speech, and Hearing Services in Schools, 49*, 938–949. https://doi.org/10.1044/2018_LSHSS-17-0159

Farquharson, K., Hogan, T. P., & Bernthal, J. E. (2017). Working memory in school-age children with and without a persistent speech sound disorder. *International Journal of Speech-Language Pathology, 20*(4), 422–433. https://doi.org/10.1080/17549507.2017.1293159

Fawcett, S., Bacsfalvi, P., & Bernhardt, B. M. (2008). Ultrasound as visual feedback in speech therapy for /r/ with adults with Down syndrome. *Down Syndrome Quarterly, 10*(1), 4–12.

Fletcher, S. G. (1992). *Articulation. A physiological approach*. Singular Publishing.

Fletcher, S. G., Dagenais, P. A., & Critz-Crosby, P. (1991). Teaching consonants to profoundly hearing-impaired speakers using palatometry. *Journal of Speech and Hearing Research, 34*, 929–942. https://doi.org/10.1044/jshr.3404.929

Flipsen, P., Jr. (2002). Longitudinal changes in articulation rate and phonetic phrase length in children with speech delay. *Journal of Speech, Language, and Hearing Research, 45*(1), 100–110. https://doi.org/10.1044/1092-4388(2002/008)

Flipsen, P., Jr. (2003). Articulation rate and speech-sound normalization failure. *Journal of Speech, Language, and Hearing Research, 46*(3), 724–737. https://doi.org/10.1044/1092-4388(2003/058)

Flipsen, P., Jr. (2014, October 10). *The problem of residual and persistent errors.* Presentation to Beaverton, Oregon, city school speech-language pathologists.

Flipsen, P., Jr. (2015). Emergence and prevalence of persistent and residual speech errors. *Seminars in Speech and Language, 36*, 217–223. https://doi.org/10.1055/s-0035-1562905

Flipsen, P., Jr. (2018, March 2). *Speech sound disorders in school age children.* Keynote presentation at the Oregon Speech-Language and Hearing Association Annual Rural Conference, Pendleton, OR.

Flipsen, P., Jr., & Sacks, S. (2015). Remediation of residual /r/ errors: A case study using the SATPAC approach. *SIG 16, Perspectives on School-Based Issues, 16* (3), 64–78. https://doi.org/10.1044/sbi16.3.64

Flipsen, P., Jr., & Sacks, S. (2017, November). *Efficacy of the SATPAC approach for treating persistent /r/ errors* [Poster presentation]. Annual convention of the American Speech-Language-Hearing Association, Los Angeles, CA.

Fucci, D. (1972). Oral vibrotactile sensation: An evaluation of normal and defective speakers. *Journal of Speech and Hearing Research, 15*, 179–184. https://doi.org/10.1044/jshr.1501.179

Fudala, J. B. (2000). *Arizona Articulation Proficiency Scale* (3rd ed.). Western Psychological Services.

Fudala, J. B., & Stegall, S. (2017). *Arizona Articulation and Phonology Scale* (4th ed.). Western Psychological Services.

Geertsema, S., & le Roux, M. (2019). The effect of blocked versus serial practice in the treatment of developmental motor-based articulation disorder. *Communication Disorders Quarterly, 40*, 1–15. https://doi.org/10.1177/1525740119836944

Gernand, K. L., & Moran, M. J. (2007). Phonological awareness abilities of 6-year-old children with mild to moderate phonological impairments. *Communication Disorders Quarterly, 28*(4), 206–215. https://doi.org/10.1177/1525740107311819

Gibbon, F. (2013, July). Bibliography of electropalatographic (EPG) studies in English. University College Cork. https://pdfs.semanticscholar.org/6aa9/ad6803435b5ed23a174309b434e13d14598d.pdf

Gibbon, F., & Lee, A. (2015). Electropalatography for older children and adults with residual speech errors. *Seminars in Speech and Language, 36*, 271–282. https://doi.org/10.1055/s-0035-1562910

Gibbon, F. E., & Paterson, L. (2006). A survey of speech and language therapists' views on electropalatography therapy outcomes in Scotland. *Child Language Teaching and Therapy, 22*, 275–292. https://doi.org/10.1191/0265659006ct308xx

Gibbon, F. E., & Wood, S. E. (2010). Visual feedback therapy with electropalatography. In A. L. Williams, S. McLeod, & R. J. McCauley (Eds.), *Interventions for speech sound disorders in children* (pp. 509–536). Paul H. Brookes Publishing.

Gick, B., Allen, B., Stavness, I., & Wilson, I. (2013). Speaking tongues are always braced. *Journal of the Acoustical Society of America, 134*, 4204. https://doi.org/10.1121/1.4831431

Gick, B., Bacsfalvi, P., Bernhardt, B. M., Oh, S., Stolar, S., & Wilson, I. (2007). A motor differentiation model for liquid substitutions: English /r/ variants in normal and disordered acquisition. *Proceedings of Meetings on Acoustics, 1*, 060003. https://doi.org/10.1121/1.2951481

Gick, B., Bernhardt, M. M., Bacsfalvi, P., & Wilson, I. (2008). Ultrasound imaging applications in second language acquisition. In J. G. H. Edwards & M. L. Zampini (Eds.), *Phonology and second language acquisition* (pp. 309–322). John Benjamins Publishing.

Gierut, J. A. (1990). Differential learning of phonological oppositions. *Journal of Speech and Hearing Research, 33*, 540–549.

Gierut, J. A. (1991). Homonymy in phonological changes. *Clinical Linguistics and Phonetics, 5*, 119–137.

Glaspey, A. (2019). *Glaspey dynamic assessment of phonology.* ATP Assessments.

Goldman, R., & Fristoe, M. (2015). *Goldman-Fristoe Test of Articulation* (3rd ed.). NCS Pearson.

Goozee, J., Murdoch, B., Ozanne, A. Cheng, Y., Hill, A., & Gibbon, F. (2007). Lingual kinematics and coordination in speech-disordered children exhibiting differentiated versus undifferentiated lingual gestures. *International Journal of Language and Communication Disorders, 42*(6), 703–724. https://doi.org/10.1080/13682820601104960

Gray, S. I., & Shelton, R. L. (1992). Self-monitoring effects on articulation carryover in school-age children. *Language, Speech, and Hearing Services in Schools, 23*, 334–342. https://doi.org/10.1044/0161-1461.2304.334

Gunther, T., & Hautvast, S. (2010). Addition of contingency management to increase home practice in young children with speech sound disorder. *International Journal of Language and Communication Disorders, 45*(3), 345–353. https://doi.org/10.3109/13682820903026762

Hagiwara, R. E. (1995). Acoustic realizations of American /R/ as produced by women and men. *UCLA Working Papers in Phonetics, 90*, 1–187.

Hayden, D. A., Namasivayam, A., K., Ward, R., Clark, A., & Eigen, J. (2021). PROMPT: A tactually grounded model. In A. L. Williams, S. McLeod, & R. J. McCauley (Eds.), *Interventions for speech sound disorders in children* (2nd ed.; pp. 477–504). Paul H. Brookes Publishing.

Heintz, J. (2015). *Buddy feedback* [Paper presentation]. Annual convention of the Texas Speech and Hearing Association, San Antonio, TX.

Helmick, J. W. (1976). Effects of therapy on articulation skills in elementary-school children. *Language, Speech, and Hearing Services in Schools, 7*, 169–172. https://doi.org/10.1044/0161-1461.0703.169

Hesketh, A. (2010). Methaphonological intervention: Phonological awareness. In A. L. Williams, S. McLeod, & R. J. McCauley (Eds.), *Interventions for speech sound disorders in children* (pp. 247–274). Paul H. Brookes Publishing.

Hesketh, A., Adams, C., Nightingale, C., & Hall, R. (2000). Phonological awareness therapy and articulatory training approaches for children with phonological disorders: A comparative study. *International Journal of Language and Communication Disorders, 35*(3), 337–354.

Hetrick, R. D., & Sommers, R. K. (1988). Unisensory and bisensory processing skills of children having misarticulations and normally speaking peers. *Journal of Speech and Hearing Research, 31,* 575–581. https://doi.org/10.1044/jshr.3104.575

Hitchcock, E. R., & Cabbage, K. (2019, November). *Biofeedback for childhood speech disorders: Practical information for clinicians* [Webinar]. Presented to American Speech-Language-Hearing Association Special Interest Groups 1, 16, and 19.

Hitchcock, E., McAllister Byun, T., & Harel, D. (2015, November). *When should we treat residual speech errors? Survey data on social, emotional, and academic impacts* [Paper presentation]. Annual convention of the American Speech-Language-Hearing Association, Denver, CO.

Hitchcock, E., McAllister Byun, T., Swartz, M., & Lazarus, R. (2017). Efficacy of electropalatography for treating misarticulations of /r/. *American Journal of Speech-Language Pathology, 26,* 1141–1158. https://doi.org/10.1044/2017_AJSLP-16-0122

Hitchcock, E. R., Swartz, M. T., & Lopez, M. (2019a). Speech sound disorders and visual biofeedback intervention: A preliminary investigation of treatment intensity. *Seminars in Speech and Language, 40,* 124–137. https://doi.org/10.1055/s-0039-1677763

Hitchcock, E. R., Swartz, M. T., & Lopez, M. (2019b, November). *Determining treatment dosage, practice conditions, and feedback methods for speech sound disorders: How do you decide?* [Seminar presentation]. Annual convention of the American Speech-Language-Hearing Association, Orlando, FL.

Hodson, B. W. (2010). *Evaluating and enhancing children's phonological systems. Research and theory to practice.* PhonoComp Publishing.

Hoffman, P. R. (1983). Interallophonic generalization of /r/ training. *Journal of Speech and Hearing Disorders, 48,* 215–221. https://doi.org/10.1044/jshd.4802.215

Hoffman, P. R., & Norris, J. A. (2010). Dynamic systems and whole-language interventions. In A. L. Williams, S. McLeod, & R. J. McCauley (Eds.), *Interventions for speech sound disorders in children* (pp. 333–354). Paul H. Brookes Publishing.

Individuals with Disabilities Education Act Amendments of 2004, PL No. 108–446, *20* U.S.C. Section 1400 et seq.

Irwin, J. V., Weston, A. J., Griffith, F. A., & Rocconi, C. (1976). Phoneme acquisition using the paired-stimuli technique in the public school setting. *Language, Speech, and Hearing Services in Schools, 7*, 220–229. https://doi.org/10.1044/0161-1461.0704.220

Jakielski, K. J., & Gildersleeve-Neumann, C. E. (2018). *Phonetic science for clinical practice.* Plural Publishing.

Jordan, L. S., Hardy, J., & Morris, H. (1978). Performance of children with good and poor articulation on tasks of tongue placement. *Journal of Speech and Hearing Research, 21*, 429–439. https://doi.org/10.1044/jshr.2103.429

Kamhi, A. G. (2006). Treatment decisions for children with speech-sound disorders. *Language, Speech, and Hearing Services in Schools, 37*, 271–279. https://doi.org/10.1044/0161-1461(2006/031)

Katz, W. F., Bharadwaj, S. V., & Carstens, B. (1999). Electromagnetic articulography treatment for an adult with Broca's aphasia and apraxia of speech. *Journal of Speech, Language, and Hearing Research, 42*, 1355–1366. https://doi.org/10.1044/jslhr.4206.1355

Katz, W. F., McNeil, M. R., & Garst, D. M. (2010). Treating apraxia of speech (AOS) with EMA-supplied visual augmented feedback. *Aphasiology, 24*(6–8), 826–837. https://doi.org/10.1080/02687030903518176

Kent, R. D. (1982). Contextual facilitation of correct speech sound production. *Language, Speech, and Hearing Services in Schools, 13*, 66–76. https://doi.org/10.1044/0161-1461.1302.66

Kent, R. D., Dembowski, J., & Lass, N. J. (1996). The acoustic characteristics of American English. In N. J. Lass (Ed.), *Principles of experimental phonetics* (pp. 185–225). Mosby.

Kim, I., LaPointe, L. L., & Stierwalt, J. A. G. (2012). The effect of feedback and practice on the acquisition of novel speech behaviors. *American Journal of Speech-Language Pathology, 21*, 89–100. https://doi.org/10.1044/1058-0360(2011/09-0082)

Klein, H. B., Grigos, M. I., McAllister Byun, T., & Davidson, L. (2012). The relationship between inexperienced listeners' perceptions and acoustic correlates of children's /r/ productions. *Clinical Linguistics and Phonetics, 26*(7), 628–645. https://doi.org/10.3109/02699206.2012.682695

Koegel, L. K., Koegel, R. L., & Ingham, J. C. (1986). Programming rapid generalization of correct articulation through self-monitoring procedures. *Journal of Speech and Hearing Disorders, 51*, 24–32. https://doi.org/10.1044/jshd.5101.24

Kuehn, D. P., & Tomblin, J. B. (1977). A cineradiography investigation of children's w/r substitutions. *Journal of Speech and Hearing Disorders, 42*, 462–473. https://doi.org/10.1044/jshd.4204.462

Ladefoged, P. (1957). Use of palatography. *Journal of Speech and Hearing Disorders, 22*(5), 764–774. https://doi.org/10.1044/jshd.2205.764

Ladefoged, P. (2005). *Vowels and consonants* (2nd ed.). Blackwell Publishers.

Ladefoged, P., & Maddieson, I. (1996). *The sounds of the world's languages.* Blackwell Publishers.

Lass, N. J., & Pannbacker, M. (2008). The application of evidence-based practice to nonspeech oral-motor treatments. *Language, Speech, and Hearing Services in Schools, 39,* 408–421. https://doi.org/10.1044/0161-1461(2008/038)

Lee, A. S. Y., & Gibbon, F. E. (2015). Non-speech oral motor treatment for children with developmental speech sound disorders. *Cochrane Database of Systematic Reviews,* (3), CD009383. https://doi.org/10.1002/14651858 .CD009383.pub2

Lee, S. A. S., Wrench, A., & Sancibrian, S. (2015). How to get started with ultrasound technology for treatment of speech sound disorders. *Perspectives on Speech Science and Orofacial Disorders, 25*(2), 66–80. https://doi .org/10.1044/ssod25.2.66

Lindau, M. (1985). The story of /r/. In V. A. Fromkin (Ed.), *Phonetic linguistics. Essays in honor of Peter Ladefoged* (pp. 157–168). Academic Press.

Locke, J. (1980). The inference of speech perception in the phonologically disordered child. Part II: Some clinically novel procedures, their use, some findings. *Journal of Speech and Hearing Disorders, 45,* 445–468. https:// doi.org/10.1044/jshd.4504.445

Lockenvitz, S., Kueker, K., & Ball, M. J. (2015). Evidence for the distinction between "consonantal-/r/" and "vocalic-/r/" in American English. *Clinical Linguistics and Phonetics, 29,* 8–10. https://doi.org/10.3109/02699206.2015 .1047962

Maas, E., Butalla, C. E., & Farinella, K. A. (2012). Feedback frequency in treatment for childhood apraxia of speech. *American Journal of Speech-Language Pathology, 21,* 239–257. https://doi.org/10.1044/1058-0360(2012/11-0119)

Maas, E., Guildersleeve-Neumann, C., Jakielski, K., Kovacs, N., Stoekel, R., Vradelis, H., & Welsh, M. (2019). Bang for your buck: A single-case experimental design study of practice amount and distribution in treatment for childhood apraxia of speech. *Journal of Speech, Language, and Hearing Research, 62,* 3160–3182. https://doi.org/10.1044/2019_JSLHR-S-18-0212

Maas, E., Robin, D. A., Austermann Hula, S. N., Freedman, S. E., Wulf, G., Ballard, K. J., & Schmidt, R. A. (2008). Principles of motor learning in treatment of motor speech disorders. *American Journal of Speech-Language Pathology, 17,* 277–298. https://doi.org/10.1044/1058-0360(2008/025)

Marchant, C. D., Shurin, P. A., Turczyk, V. A., Wasikowski, D. E., Tutihasi, M. A., & Kinney, S. E. (1984). Course and outcome of otitis media in early infancy: A prospective study. *Journal of Pediatrics, 104*(6), 826–831.

Mason, R. (1982). *Oral facial examination in speech pathology* [VHS Video]. Continuing education presentation at Purdue University, West Lafayette, IN.

McAllister, T., Preston, J. L., Hitchcock, E. R., & Hill, J. (2020). Protocol for correcting residual errors with spectral, ultrasound, traditional speech therapy randomized controlled trial (C-RESULTS RCT). *BMC Pediatrics, 20,* 66. https://doi.org/10.1186/s12887-020-1941-5

McAllister Byun, T., & Campbell, H. (2016). Differential effects of visual-acoustic biofeedback intervention for residual speech errors. *Frontiers in Neuroscience, 10*(567), 1–11. https://doi.org/10.3389/fnhum.2016.00567

McAllister Byun, T., & Hitchcock, E. R. (2012). Investigating the use of traditional and spectral feedback for approaches to intervention for /r/ misarticulation. *American Journal of Speech-Language Pathology*, *21*, 207–221. https://doi.org/10.1044/1058-0360(2012/11-0083)

McAllister Byun, T., Hitchcock, E. R., & Swartz, M. T. (2014). Retroflex versus bunched in treatment for rhotic misarticulation: Evidence from ultrasound biofeedback intervention. *Journal of Speech, Language, and Hearing Research*, *57*, 2116–2130. https://doi.org/10.1044/2014_JSLHR-S-14-0034

McAllister Byun, T., Swartz, M. T., Halpin, P. F., Szeredi, D., & Maas, E. (2016). Direction of attentional focus in biofeedback treatment for /r/ misarticulation. *International Journal of Language and Communication Disorders*, *51*(4), 384–401. https://doi.org/10.1111/1460-6984.12215

McCormack, J., Harrison, L. J., McLeod, S., & McAllister, L. (2011). A nationally representative study of the association between communication impairments at 4–5 years and children's life activities at 7–9 years. *Journal of Speech, Language, and Hearing Research*, *54*, 1328–1348. https://doi.org/10.1044/1092-4388(2011/10-0155)

McDonald, E. T. (1964). *Articulation testing and treatment: A sensory motor approach*. Stanwix House.

McLeod, S., & Arciuli, J. (2009). School-aged children's production of /s/ and /r/ consonant clusters. *Folia Phoniatrica et Logopaedica*, *61*, 336–341. https://doi.org/10.1159/000252850

McLeod, S., & Searl, J. (2006). Adaptation to an electropalatograph palate: Acoustic, impressionistic, and perceptual data. *American Journal of Speech-Language Pathology*, *15*, 192–206. https://doi.org/10.1044/1058-0360 (2006/018)

McLeod, S., & Singh, S. (2009). *Seeing speech. A quick guide to speech sounds*. Plural Publishing.

McNutt, J. C. (1977). Oral sensory and motor behaviors of children with /s/ or /r/ misarticulations. *Journal of Speech and Hearing Research*, *20*, 694–703. https://doi.org/10.1044/jshr.2101.192

McReynolds, L. V. (1972). Articulation generalization during articulation training. *Language and Speech*, *15*(2), 149–155.

Melby-Lervag, M., Halaas Lyster, S-A., & Hulme, C. (2012). Phonological skills and their role in learning to read: A meta-analytic review. *Psychological Bulletin*, *138*(2), 322–352. https://doi.org/10.1037/a0026744

Miccio, A. W. (2002). Clinical problem solving: Assessment of phonological disorders. *American Journal of Speech-Language Pathology*, *11*, 221–229. https://doi.org/10.1044/1058-0360(2002/023)

Mielke, J., Baker, A., & Archangeli, D. (2016). Individual-level contact limits phonological complexity; Evidence from bunched and retroflex /ɹ/. *Language*, *92*, 101–140. https://doi.org/10.1353/lan.2016.0019

Mines, M. A., Hanson, B. F., & Shoup, J. E. (1978). Frequency of occurrence of phonemes in conversational English. *Language and Speech*, *21*(3), 221–241.

Mullen, R., & Schooling, T. (2010). The national outcomes measurement system for pediatric speech-language pathology. *Language, Speech, and Hearing Services in Schools, 41*, 44–60. https://doi.org/10.1044/0161-1461(2009/08-0051)

Neal, A. (2020). */r/ Therapy–Part 1* [Webinar]. Speechpathology.com. https://www.speechpathology.com/slp-ceus/course/r-therapy-part-1-9523

Neel, A. T. (2010). Using acoustic phonetics in clinical practice. *Perspectives on Speech Science and Orofacial Disorders, 20*(1), 14–24. https://doi.org/10.1044/ssod20.1.14

OSERS (Office of Special Education and Rehabilitative Services). (2007, March 8). Letter to ASHA regarding "adversely affects educational performance." https://www.asha.org/siteassets/uploadedfiles/advocacy/federal/idea/OSEPResponseLetterGuidance.pdf

Overstake, C. P. (1976). Investigation of the efficacy of a treatment program for deviant swallowing and allied problems. *International Journal of Oral Myology, 2*, 1–6.

Pearson, B. Z., Velleman, S. L., Bryant, T. J., & Charko, T. (2009). Phonological milestones for African American English-speaking children learning mainstream American English as a second dialect. *Language, Speech, and Hearing Services in Schools, 40*(3), 229–244. https://doi.org/10.1044/0161-1461(2008/08-0064)

Potter, R. K., Kopp, G. A., & Green, H. A. (1947). *Visible speech*. D. Van Nostrand.

Potter. S. O. L. (1882). *Speech and its defects*. Blakiston, Son & Co.

Prather, E. M., Hedrick, D. L., & Kern, C. A. (1975). Articulation development in children aged two to four years. *Journal of Speech and Hearing Disorders, 40*(2), 179–191. https://doi.org/10.1044/jshd.4002.179

Preston, J. L., Brick, N., & Landi, N. (2013). Ultrasound biofeedback treatment for persisting childhood apraxia of speech. *American Journal of Speech-Language Pathology, 22*(4), 627–643. https://doi.org/10.1044/1058-0360(2013/12-0139)

Preston, J. L., & Edwards, M. L. (2007). Phonological processing skill of adolescents with residual speech sound errors. *Language, Speech, and Hearing Services in Schools, 38*, 297–308. https://doi.org/10.1044/0161-1461(2007/032)

Preston, J. L., Hitchcock, E. R., & Leece, M. C. (2020). Auditory perception and ultrasound biofeedback treatment outcomes for children with residual /ɹ/ distortions: A randomized control trial. *Journal of Speech, Language, and Hearing Research, 63*, 444–455. https://doi.org/10.1044/2019_JSLHR-19-00060

Preston, J., & Leece, M. (2019, November). *Treating /r/ errors: Cueing and practice strategies informed by evidence* [Seminar presentation]. Annual convention of the American Speech-Language-Hearing Association, Orlando, FL.

Preston, J. L., & Leece, M. C. (2021). Articulation interventions. In A. L. Williams, S. McLeod, & R. J. McCauley (Eds.), *Interventions for speech sound disorders in children* (2nd ed., pp. 419–445). Paul H. Brookes Publishing.

Preston, J. L., Leece, M. C., & Maas, E. (2017). Motor-based treatment with and without ultrasound feedback for residual speech-sound errors. *International Journal of Language and Communication Disorders, 52*(1), 80–94. https://doi.org/10.1111/1460-6984.12259

Preston, J. L., Leece, M. C., & Storto, J. (2019). Tutorial: Speech motor chaining treatment for school-age children with speech sound disorders. *Language, Speech, and Hearing Services in Schools, 50*, 343–355. https://doi.org/10.1044/2018_LSHSS-18-0081

Preston, J. L., Maas, E., Whittle, J., Leece, M. C., & McCabe, P. (2016). Limited acquisition and generalization of rhotics with ultrasound visual feedback in childhood apraxia. *Clinical Linguistics and Phonetics, 30*(3–5), 363–381. https://doi.org/10.3109/02699206.2015.1052563

Radulovic, J., Jovasevic, V., & Meyer, M. A. A. (2017). Neurobiological mechanisms of state-dependent learning. *Current Opinion in Neurobiology, 45*, 92–98. https://doi.org/10.1016/j.conb.2017.05.013

Ringel, R., & Ewanowski, S. (1965). Oral perception: 1. Two-point discrimination. *Journal of Speech and Hearing Research, 8*, 389–400. https://doi.org/10.1044/jshr.0804.389

Ringel, R., House, A. S., Burk, K. W., Dolinsky, J. P., & Scott, C. M. (1970). Some relations between orosensory discrimination and articulatory aspects of speech production. *Journal of Speech and Hearing Disorders, 35*, 3–11. https://doi.org/10.1044/jshd.3501.03

Ristuccia, C. (2002). *The Entire World of R. Instructional workbook. A phonemic approach to /r/ remediation.* Say It Right.

Rogers, G. (2011, November). *Parent effectiveness in treating speech sound disorders through tactile biofeedback* [Poster presentation]. Annual convention of the American Speech-Language-Hearing Association, San Diego, CA.

Rogers, G. (2013). Hand-held tactile biofeedback as a cuing mechanism to elicit and generalize correct /R/: A case study. *eHearsay: Electronic Journal of the Ohio Speech-Language Hearing Association, 3*(2), 39–55.

Rogers, G., & Chesin, M. (2013). Examining the clinical application of intra-oral tactile biofeedback in short-duration therapy targeting misarticulated /s/. *PSHA Journal, 2013*, 5–18.

Rogers, G., Lee, J., & Parmentier, E. (2012, November). *Examining the effectiveness of tactile biofeedback in charter schools* [Poster presentation]. Annual convention of the American Speech-Language-Hearing Association, Atlanta, GA.

Ruscello, D. M. (1975). The importance of word position in articulation therapy. *Language, Speech, and Hearing Services in Schools, 6*, 190–196. https://doi.org/10.1044/0161-1461.0604.190

Ruscello, D. M. (1995a). Visual feedback in treatment of residual phonological disorders. *Journal of Communication Disorders, 28*, 279–302.

Ruscello, D. M. (1995b). Speech appliances in the treatment of phonological disorders. *Journal of Communication Disorders, 28*, 331–353.

Rusiewicz, H. L., & Riveria, J. L. (2017). The effect of hand gesture cues within the treatment of /r/ for a college-aged adult with persisting childhood apraxia of speech. *American Journal of Speech-Language Pathology, 26,* 1236 1243. https://doi.org/10.1044/2017_AJSLP-15-0172

Rvachew, S., & Brosseau-Lapré, F. (2015). A randomized trial of 12-week interventions for the treatment of developmental phonological disorder in Francophone children. *American Journal of Speech-Language Pathology, 24*(4), 637–658. https://doi.org/10.1044/2015_AJSLP-14-0056

Rvachew, S., & Herbay, A. (2017). *Speech Assessment and Interactive Learning System* (SAILS, v. 1.0). https://apps.apple.com/ca/app/sails/id1207583276

Rvachew, S., & Nowak, M. (2001). The effect of target-selection strategy on phonological learning. *Journal of Speech, Language, and Hearing Research, 44,* 610–623.

Saben, C. B., & Ingham, J. C. (1991). The effects of minimal pairs treatment on the speech-sound production of two children with phonologic disorders. *Journal of Speech and Hearing Research, 34,* 1023–1040. https://doi.org/10.1044/jshr.3405.1023

Sacks, S. (2017, November). *Using the SATPAC program and approach with middle school students with highly unintelligible speech* [Seminar presentation]. Annual convention of the American-Speech-Language-Hearing Association, Los Angeles, CA.

Sacks, S., & Flipsen, P., Jr. (2013, November). *Efficacy of the SATPAC approach for remediating persistent /s/ errors* [Seminar presentation]. Annual convention of the American-Speech-Language-Hearing Association, Chicago, IL.

Sacks, S., Flipsen, P., Jr., & Neils-Strunjas, J. (2013). Effectiveness of Systematic Articulation Training Program Accessing Computers (SATPAC) approach to remediate dentalized and interdental /s,z/: A preliminary study. *Perceptual and Motor Skills: Perception, 117*(2), 559–577. https://doi.org/10.2466/24.10.PMS.117x21z2

Sander, E. K. (1972). When are speech sounds learned? *Journal of Speech and Hearing Disorders, 37,* 55–63. https://doi.org/10.1044/jshd.3701.55

Schmidt, A. M. (2007). Evaluating a new clinical palatometry system. *Advances in Speech-Language Pathology, 9*(1), 73–81. https://doi.org/10.1080/14417040601123650

Schmidt, R. A., & Lee, T. D. (2005). *Motor control and learning. A behavioral emphasis* (4th ed.). Human Kinetics.

Secord, W. A., Boyce, S. E., Donahue, J. S., Fox, R. A., & Shine, R. E. (2007). *Eliciting sounds. Techniques and strategies for clinicians* (2nd ed.). Thomson Delmar Learning.

Shawker, T. H., & Sonies, B. C. (1985). Ultrasound biofeedback for speech training. Instrumentation and preliminary results. *Investigative Radiology, 20,* 90–93.

Shriberg, L. D. (1975). A response evocation program for /ɝ/. *Journal of Speech and Hearing Disorders, 40,* 92–105. https://doi.org/10.1044/jshd.4001.92

Shriberg, L. D. (1980). An intervention procedure for children with persistent /r/ errors. *Language, Speech, and Hearing Services in Schools, 11*, 102–110. https://doi.org/10.1044/0161-1461.1102.102

Shriberg, L. D. (1982). Diagnostic assessment of developmental phonological disorders. The rhotacist and the Maytag repair man. In M. Crary (Ed.), *Phonological intervention: Concepts and procedures* (pp. 35–60). College-Hill Press.

Shriberg, L. D. (2010). Childhood speech sound disorders: From postbehaviorism to the postgenomic era. In R. Paul & P. Flipsen Jr. (Eds.), *Speech sound disorders: In honor of Lawrence D. Shriberg* (pp. 1–33). Plural Publishing.

Shriberg, L. D., Flipsen, P., Jr., Karlsson, H. B., & McSweeny, J. L. (2001). Acoustic phenotypes for speech-genetics studies: An acoustic marker for residual /ɚ/ distortions. *Clinical Linguistics and Phonetics, 15*, 631–650. https://doi.org/10.1080/02699200110069429

Shriberg, L. D., Friel-Patti, S., Flipsen, P., Jr., & Brown, R. L. (2000). Otitis media, fluctuant hearing loss, and speech-language outcomes: A preliminary structural equation model. *Journal of Speech, Language, and Hearing Research, 43*, 100–120. https://doi.org/10.1044/jslhr.4301.100

Shriberg, L. D., Kent, R. D., McAllister, T., & Preston, J. L. (2019). *Clinical phonetics* (5th ed.). Pearson.

Shuster, L. I. (1998). The perception of correctly and incorrectly produced /r/. *Journal of Speech, Language, and Hearing Research, 41*, 941–950. https://doi.org/10.1044/jslhr.4104.941

Shuster, L. I., Ruscello, D. M., & Smith, K. D. (1992). Evoking [r] using visual feedback. *American Journal of Speech-Language Pathology, 1*(2), 29–34. https://doi.org/10.1044/1058-0360.0103.29

Shuster, L. I., Ruscello, D. M., & Toth, A. R. (1995). The use of visual feedback to elicit correct /r/. *American Journal of Speech-Language Pathology, 4*(2), 37–44. https://doi.org/10.1044/1058-0360.0402.37

Silverman, F. H., & Paulus, P. G. (1989). Peer reactions to teenagers who substitute /w/ for /r/. *Language, Speech, and Hearing Services in Schools, 20*, 219–221. https://doi.org/10.1044/0161-1461.2002.219

Skelton, S. L. (2004). Concurrent task sequencing in single-phoneme phonologic treatment and generalization. *Journal of Communication Disorders, 37*, 131–155. https://doi.org/10.1016/j.jcomdis.2003.08.002

Skelton, S. L., & Funk, T. E. (2004). Teaching speech sounds to young children using randomly ordered, variable complex task sequences. *Perceptual and Motor Skills, 99*, 602–604. https://doi.org/10.2466/pms.99.2.602-604

Skelton, S. L., & Hagopian, A. L. (2014). Using randomized variable practice in the treatment of childhood apraxia of speech. *American Journal of Speech-Language Pathology, 23*, 599–611. https://doi.org/10.1044/2014_AJSLP-12-0169

Skelton, S. L., & Kerber, J. R. (2005, November). *Using concurrent treatment to teach multiple phonemes to phonologically disordered children* [Poster presentation]. Annual convention of the American Speech-Language-Hearing Association, San Diego, CA.

Skelton, S. L., & Price, J. R. (2006, November). *A preliminary comparison of concurrent and traditional speech-sound treatments* [Seminar presentation]. Annual convention of the American Speech-Language-Hearing Association, Miami, FL.

Skelton, S. L., & Resciniti, D. N. (2009, November). *Using a motor learning treatment with phonologically disordered children* [Poster presentation]. Annual convention of the American Speech-Language-Hearing Association, New Orleans, LA.

Skelton, S. L., & Richard, J. T. (2016). Application of a motor learning treatment for speech sound disorders in small groups. *Perceptual and Motor Skills*, *122*(3), 840–854. https://doi.org/10.1177/0031512516647693

Skelton, S. L., & Snell, S. (2014, November). *The efficacy of concurrent treatment as a motor-skill approach for childhood apraxia of speech* [Poster presentation]. Annual convention of the American Speech-Language-Hearing Association, Orlando, FL.

Smit, A. B. (1986). Ages of speech sound acquisition: Comparisons and critiques of several normative studies. *Language, Speech, and Hearing Services in Schools*, *17*, 175–186. https://doi.org/10.1044/0161-1461.1703.175

Smit, A. B. (1993). Phonologic error distributions in the Iowa-Nebraska articulation norms project: Consonant singletons. *Journal of Speech and Hearing Research*, *36*, 533–547. https://doi.org/10.1044/jshr.3605.931

Smit, A. B., Hand, L., Freilinger, J. J., Bernthal, J. E., & Bird, A. (1990). The Iowa articulation norms project and its Nebraska replication. *Journal of Speech and Hearing Disorders*, *55*, 779–798. https://doi.org/10.1044/jshr.3402.446

Sommers, R. K., Leiss, R. H., Delp, M. A., Gerber, A. J., Fundrella, D., Smith II, R. M., Revucky, M. V., Ellis, D., & Haley, V. (1967). Factors related to the effectiveness of articulation therapy for kindergarten, first, and second grade children. *Journal of Speech and Hearing Research*, *10*, 428–437. https://doi.org/10.1044/jshr.1003.428

Speirs, R. L., & Maktabi, M. A. (1990). Tongue skills and clearance of toffee in two age-groups and in children with problems of speech articulation. *Journal of Dentistry for Children*, *57*, 356–360.

Steinberg Lowe, M., & Buchwald, A. (2017). The impact of feedback frequency on performance in a novel speech motor learning task. *Journal of Speech, Language, and Hearing Research*, *60*, 1712–1725. https://doi.org/10.1044/2017_JSLHR-S-16-0207

Stone, M. (1990). A three-dimensional model of tongue movement based on ultrasound and x-ray microbeam data. *Journal of the Acoustical Society of America*, *87*, 2207–2217. https://doi.org/10.1121/1.399188

Stone, M. (2005). A guide to analysing tongue motion from ultrasound images. *Clinical Linguistics and Phonetics*, *19*(6–7), 455–501. https://doi.org/10.1080/02699200500113558

Storkel, H. L. (2018). The complexity approach to phonological treatment: How to select treatment targets. *Language, Speech, and Hearing Services in Schools*, *49*, 463–481. https://doi.org/10.1044/2017_LSHSS-17-0082

Sugden, E., Baker, E., Munro, N., Williams, A. L., & Trivette, C. M. (2018). Service delivery and intervention intensity for phonology-based speech sound disorders. *International Journal of Language and Communication Disorders, 53*(4), 718–734. https://doi.org/10.1111/1460-6984.12399

Sugden, E., Lloyd, S., Lam, J., & Cleland, J. (2019). Systematic review of ultrasound biofeedback in intervention for speech sound disorders. *International Journal of Language and Communication Disorders, 54*(5), 705–728. https://doi.org/10.1111/1460-6984.12478

Templin, M. C. (1957). *Certain language skills in children.* University of Minnesota, The Institute of Child Welfare.

Thomas, J. L. (2016). Decoding eligibility under the IDEA: Interpretations of "adversely affect educational performance." *Campbell Law Review, 38*(1), 72–107.

Travis, L. E. (1931). *Speech pathology.* D. Appleton and Company.

Trulsson, M., & Essick, G. K. (1997). Low-threshold mechanoreceptive afferents in the human lingual nerve. *Journal of Neurophysiology, 77,* 737–748.

University of Iowa Research Foundation. (2016). *Sounds of speech.* https://apps.apple.com/us/app/sounds-of-speech/id780656219

Van Riper, C. (1939). *Speech correction. Principles and methods.* Prentice Hall.

Van Riper, C. (1954). *Speech correction. Principles and methods* (3rd ed.). Prentice Hall.

Van Riper, C., & Erickson, R. L. (1996). *Speech correction. An introduction of speech pathology and audiology* (9th ed.). Allyn & Bacon.

Weaver-Spurlock, S., & Brasseur, J. (1988). The effects of simultaneous sound-position training on the generalization of [s]. *Language, Speech, and Hearing Services in Schools, 19,* 259–271. https://doi.org/10.1044/0161-1461.1903.259

Weinberg, B., Liss, G. M., & Hillis, J. (1970). A comparative study of visual, manual, and oral form identification in speech impaired and normal speaking children. In J. F. Bosma (Ed.), *Second symposium on oral sensation and perception* (pp. 350–356). Charles Thomas.

Wellman, B., Case, I., Mengert, I., & Bradbury, D. (1931). Speech sounds of young children. *University of Iowa Studies in Child Welfare, 5*(2). University of Iowa Child Welfare Research Station.

Westbury, J. R., Hashi, M., & Lindstrom, M. J. (1998). Differences among speakers in lingual articulation for American English /ɹ/. *Speech Communication, 26,* 203–226. https://doi.org/10.1016/S0167-6393(98)00058-2

Williams, A. L. (2012). Intensity in phonological intervention: Is there a prescribed amount? *International Journal of Speech-Language Pathology, 14*(5), 456–461. https://doi.org/10.3109/17549507.2012.688866

Wolfe, V., Presley, C., & Mesaris, J. (2003). The importance of sound identification training in phonological intervention. *American Journal of Speech-Language Pathology, 12,* 282–288. https://doi.org/10.1044/1058-0360(2003/074)

Wong, A. W.-K., Whitehill, T. L., Ma, E. P.-M., & Masters, R. (2013). Effects of practice schedules on speech motor learning. *International Journal of*

Speech-Language Pathology, 15(5), 511–523. https://doi.org/10.3109/1754 9507.2012.761282

Woodcock, R. W., Camarata, S., & Camarata, M. (2019). *Woodcock-Camarata Articulation Battery (WCAB)*. Schoolhouse Educational Services.

Wulf, G., & Shea, C. H. (2004). Understanding the role of augmented feedback. The good, the bad, and the ugly. In A. M. Williams & N. J. Hodges (Eds.), *Skill acquisition in sport: Research, theory, and practice* (pp. 121–144). Taylor & Francis.

Index

Note: Page numbers in **bold** reference non-text material.

A

Academic failure, as criteria for speech services, 7
Accuracy assessment, of /r/ production, 57–59, 68–71, 139
Acoustic analysis, 13
Acoustic feedback, visual. *See* Visual acoustic feedback
Aerodynamic analysis, 13
Alveolar consonants, 121
American English, /r/ production in, 19, 21–22
American Speech-Language-Hearing Association
  academic failure as speech treatment criteria, 7
  levels of evidence, 17, **17**
Amplified auditory stimulation, 76, **77**
Ankyloglossia, 51
Approximant, /r/ as, 3, 19
Articulate Instruments, 195
Articulation therapy
  current approach to, 107–108
  description of, 79–88
  traditional
    advantages of, **198**
    bottom-up approach, 129–130
    concurrent treatment, 129–136, **134–135**, 139, **198**
    dimensions of, 102
    disadvantages of, **198**
    ear training, 105–106, 108

evidence to support, 108–112, **113**
homework in, 93–94, 111
modifications in, 123
nonsense material, 106
/r/ elicitation, 114–119
randomized treatment sequence in, 130, **131–132**
reconfiguration, 107
self-monitoring in, 110–111, 122–123
summary of, **112**
treatment hierarchy, 129
treatment sequence, 102, **103–104**, 112, **113**, 123
Van Riper's approach, 102, 104–110, 122–123
visual input and, 156
Articulators, 148
Artificial palate, 9, 11
ASHA. *See* American Speech-Language-Hearing Association
Auditory feedback, 144–145
Auditory stimulation, 115
Automaticity, 90–91, 137

B

Bad habit, /r/ errors as, 4, 39
Bias, 16
Bite block, 120–121, **122**
Bite stick, 120–121
Bostonian dialect, 49

Bullying, 6
Bunched /r/, 116–118
Bunched tongue shape, 20, 23–26, **25**, **84**, 116–117

C

Case history, 49
"Challenge point," 88–89
Childhood apraxia, 52, 185
Clear speech, 29
Coarticulation, 29, 114
CompleteSpeech, 165
Comprehension skills, 50
Computerized Speech Lab system, 182
Concurrent treatment, 129–136, **134–135**, 139, **198**
Consonants
    alveolar, 121
    cluster of, 35, 37, **38**
    description of, 19
    glide, 44
    /r/ as, 14, **15**, 35, 37
    singletons, 35, **36–37**
    stop, 114
Constriction
    gender differences in, 21–22
    lip, 20, 127
    oral cavity, 20, 22, 127
    pharyngeal cavity, 20, 22
    pharynx, 4, 20, 116
    /r/ production, 20–21
    ultrasound studies of, 21

D

Derhotacized /r/, 43, 49
Developmental logic
    alternatives to, 37, 39–41
    description of, 33, 52
Diadochokinetic rate tasks, 52
Dialects, 6, 49
Discrimination drill, for perceptual therapy, 75–76
Discrimination training, in speech sound therapy, 45
Down syndrome, 186

Dynamic palatography, 9, 11
Dynamic palatometry, 9

E

Ear infections, 49
Ear training, 105–106, 108
Electromagnetic articulography
    description of, 14
    tongue bracing studies using, 27
Electropalatography
    advantages of, 165, **198**
    age limitations for, 199
    basics of, 158–159
    components of, 159
    cost constraints of, 197
    definition of, 9
    description of, viii
    disadvantages of, 165, 167, **198**
    duration of therapy, 162
    elements of, 9, **10**
    equipment manufacturers for, 165
    establishment and stabilization with, 162–164
    limitations of, 11
    on-screen image, 159, **160–161**
    orientation to, 162, **163**
    pseudopalates in, 9, 11, 158, **160**
    remediation uses of, 164–167, **166**
    split-screen presentation in, 159
    studies of, 164–165, **166**
    tongue bracing studies using, 27, **28**
    training palate in, 159
Eliciting Sounds (Secord), 114
EMA. *See* Electromagnetic articulography
English as a second language learners, 186
EPG. *See* Electropalatography
Evidence-based practice
    description of, ix, 16, 105
    elements of, 16–18
    levels of evidence, 17, **17**
    progress tracking, 58
    summary of, 18, **18**
External feedback
    description of, 143–144
    verbal feedback. *See* Verbal feedback

visual feedback. *See* Visual acoustic feedback; Visual feedback
External focus, 83

F

F1, 173
F2, 173
F3, 173
F4, 173
Facilitating contexts, 114–115
Feedback
    alternative, 121–122
    auditory, 144–145
    challenge point and, 89
    external, 143–144
    general type of, 83–84
    internal, 144–145
    kinesthetic, 145
    knowledge of performance, 83–85, **84**, 144, 147–148, 157, 170, 187
    knowledge of results, 83–85, **84**, 144, 147, 157, 170, 187
    in motor learning, 83–86
    proprioceptive, 144–145
    quantity of, 85, 143
    in /r/ production, 52
    tactile. *See* Tactile feedback
    timing of, 85–86, 143
    ultrasound. *See* Ultrasound
    verbal, 143–144
    visual. *See* Visual feedback
    visual acoustic. *See* Visual acoustic feedback
Fiberoptic endoscopy, 13
Fletcher, Samuel, 9
Formant frequencies, 172

G

Gender
    constriction differences, 21–22
    oral cavity differences, 5, 21–22
    pharyngeal cavity differences, 5, 21–22
    r mastery and, 37
    speech sound differences based on, 21–22
    vocal tract differences, 5, 21

General feedback type, 83–84
Generalization
    description of, 89–90
    failure of, 90
    measurement of, 90
    motor learning principles and, 90
    self-assessment, 91
    self-monitoring, 91–92
Gestural cues, 119
Glide consonant, 44
Goldilocks Zone, 88

H

Hearing acuity assessments, 50
Hearing impairment, 185
Hodson, Barbara, 74, 76
Homework, 93–94, 111

I

IDEA. *See* Individuals with Disabilities Education Act
Individuals with Disabilities Education Act, 7
Instrumental approaches, 94
Internal feedback, 144–145
Internal focus, 83
International Phonetic Association, 14
Intraoral appliance, removable, 153–154
Ionizing radiation, 11
IPA. *See* International Phonetic Association

J

Jaw aperture, 127
Jaw stabilization, 119–121, 137
Judgment tasks, for perception therapy, 74

K

Kinesthetic feedback, 145
Knowledge of performance feedback, 83–85, **84**, 144, 147–148, 157, 170, 187

Knowledge of results feedback, 83–85, **84**, 144, 147, 157, 170, 187
KP. *See* Knowledge of performance
KR. *See* Knowledge of results

L

/l/, 117, 178
Language comprehension, 50–51
Late Eight, The (Bleile), 114
Levels of evidence, 17, **17**
Linear predictive coding, 13, 173, 175, **176**
Lips
    constriction of, 20, 127
    rounding of, 20
Liquid consonant, /r/ as, 19, 26
Liquid gliding, 48
LPC. *See* Linear predictive coding

M

Mason, Robert, 52
Mastery of /r/
    age for, 35, **36**, 37
    in consonant clusters, 35, 37, **38**
    defining of, 34–35
    as singletons, 35, **36–37**
McDonald, Eugene, 114
Metaphon, 78
Metaphors, 118
Middle ear infections, 49, 74
Minimal pairs therapy, 77–78
Mirrors, 156
Molars, 52
Motivation, 105
Motor learning
    description of, 30
    principles of, 79–80, 86–88, 147
    progress form for, 96–99
Motor skills, 52–53
Motor theory of speech perception, 5
Multimedia Speech Pathology, 182

N

Naturalistic intervention, ix
New York dialect, 49

Nonspeech oral motor exercises, 94–95, 119
Nucleus situations, 94

O

Older children, /r/ errors in, 5–8
OMDs. *See* Oromyofunctional disorders
Oral cavity
    constriction/narrowing of, 20, 22, 127
    gender differences in, 5, 21
Oral-facial examination, 51–52
Oromyofunctional disorders, 53

P

Palate
    artificial, 9, 11
    narrow, 51
    pseudopalate, 9, 11, 158, **160**
    structure of, 51–52
Palatography
    description of, 8–11
    dynamic, 9, 11
    electropalatography. *See* Electropalatography
    static, 9
Parents, 93
PENTAX Medical, 182
Perceptual problems
    identification of, 54–56, 199
    /r/ errors as, 4–5, 45–47, 54–56
    same–different task for, 54–55
    Speech Production–Perception Task for, 55–56, 63–67, 74
Perceptual therapy, 73–76, **75**, 106
Persistent errors, 39, **39**, 44, 90
Perturbation theory, 21
Pharyngeal cavity
    constriction in, 20, 22
    gender differences in, 5, 21–22
Pharyngeal constriction, 4, 20, 116
Phoneme blending tasks, 78
Phoneme segmentation tasks, 78
Phoneme sorting tasks, 78
Phonetic placement procedures, 116–117, 156

Phonetic symbols, 14, **15**
Phonological awareness activities, 78
Phonological pattern analysis, 48
Phonological problems
    definition of, 47
    identification of, 56–57, 199
    /r/ errors as, 47–48, 53
Phonological therapy, 76–78
Phonological working memory, 48
Posny, Alexa, 7
Potter, Samuel, vii
Praat, 182
Practice-based evidence, 17
Preston, Jonathan, 45
Progress tracking, 58, 96–99
PROMPT, x
Pronunciation Coach, 117
Proprioceptive feedback, 144–145
Pseudopalates, 9, 11, 158, **160**

Q

Quality of life, 6

R

/r/
    acoustic analysis of, 13
    in American English, 19, 21–23
    as approximant, 3, 19
    articulatory features of, 19–22
    bunched, 116–118
    challenges associated with, 2–5
    as consonant, 14, **15**
    constrictions for, 20–22. *See also*
        Constriction
    contextual differences, 29, **29**
    definition of, 172
    derhotacized, 43, 49
    different types of, 27–31
    elicitation of, 114–119, 124–127
    facilitating contexts for, 114–115
    historical studies of, vii
    imitation of, 115
    as liquid consonant, 19, 26
    mastery of
        age for, 35, **36**, 37
        in consonant clusters, 35, 37, **38**

    defining of, 34–35
    as singletons, 35, **36–37**
    modeling of, 115–116, **116**
    motor learning for, 30
    palatography studies of, 8–11, **10**
    phonetic placement procedures for
        eliciting, 116–117, 124–127
    phonetic symbols for, 14, **15**
    remediation of. *See* Remediation
    removable intraoral appliance,
        153–154
    as resonant sound, 172
    retroflex, 117–118, 124–125
    shaping of, from /l/, 117, 178
    singletons, 35, **36–37**, 57
    tongue shapes for production of,
        3, 22–26, **25**. *See also* Tongue
        shapes
    touch cues for, 118
    treatment of. *See* Remediation
    as trilled sound, 14
    ultrasound studies of, 11–13, **12**. *See
        also* Ultrasound
    versions of, 4, 27–31
    vocal tract narrowing for production
        of, 3
    as vowel, 14, **15**
    [w] substitution for. *See* [w]
        substitution
    word chains for, 87
    x-ray studies of, 11
/r/ assessments
    case history, 49
    dialect, 49
    hearing acuity, 50
    language comprehension, 50–51
    motor skills, 52–53
    oral-facial examination, 51–52
    palate structure, 51–52
    stimulability, 50, 53–54, 61–62
    structural issues, 51–52
    tongue growth patterns, 52
    tonsil enlargement, 51
/r/ distortion
    age of onset, 43
    in American dialects, 6, 49
    description of, vii–viii
    dialects and, 6, 49

/r/ distortion *(continued)*
  as persistent error, 39, **39**, 44, 90
  in preschoolers, 43
  as residual error, 39, **39**, 44
  [w] substitution for /r/ versus,
    44–45, 47
/r/ errors
  in adults, 1–2
  articulation therapy for, ix
  as bad habit, 4, 39
  bullying because of, 6
  clinician-related factors for, 3–4
  diagnosis of, 53–57
  in females, 2
  interventions for. *See* Remediation
  job prospects affected by, 6
  lack of concern about, 5–6
  natural history of, 6
  non-interventional resolution of, 6,
    18
  in older children, 5–8
  as perceptual problem, 4–5, 45–47,
    54–56
  as phonological problem, 47–48, 53
  prognosis for, viii
  quality of life affected by, 6
  reasons for not correcting, 5–6
  scope of, 1–2
  stimulability of, 50
  success rate for, 1–2
  tactile sensitivity in, 145–146
  target-related factors for, 2–3
  therapy-related factors for, 4–5
  tongue-tie with, 51
  tonsil enlargement with, 51
  ultrasound applications, 185–186
  visual acoustic feedback for, 179,
    180–181
  [w] substitution versus, 43–44
  watch-and-see approach for, 40
/r/ production
  accuracy assessments, 57–59, 68–71,
    139
  consistency assessments, 59
  cues for, 118–119, 127
  feedback during, 52
  generalization tests, 57, **58**
  gestural cues for, 119

  homework for, 93–94
  metaphors used in, 118
  tactile feedback during, 144, 154
  tongue contact with vocal tract
    during, 26–27, **28**, 145
  touch cues for, 118
Reconfiguration, 107
Reductionism, 129
Remediation
  age of onset, 4
  articulation therapy. *See* Articulation
    therapy
  automaticity in, 90–91
  child's agreement to, 18, 105
  concurrent, 129–136, **134–135**, 139,
    198
  developmental logic for, 33, 37,
    39–41, 52
  efficiency of, 89
  jaw stabilization for, 119–121, 137
  justification for, 5
  motor learning principles, 79–80,
    86–88
  nonspeech oral motor exercises,
    94–95
  normative data, 34–37
  in older children, 7–8
  perceptual therapy, 73–76, **75**
  phonological therapy, 76–78
  problem-focused approach to, 199
  progress in, 88–89, 96–99
  removable intraoral appliance,
    153–154
  Speech Buddies, 121, 148–153, **149**,
    151–152, 154, 169, 197, **198**
  Systematic Articulation Training
    Program Accessing Computers.
    See Systematic Articulation
    Training Program Accessing
    Computers
  tactile feedback, 143–148
  timing of, 33–41
  ultrasound. *See* Ultrasound
  visual acoustic feedback. *See* Visual
    acoustic feedback
Removable intraoral appliance, 153–154
Residual errors, 39, **39**, 44
Resonant sound, 172

Retroflex /r/, 117–118, 124–125
Retroflex tongue shape, 3, 20, 23–26, **25**, **84**, 117
Rhotacism, vii
Rhotic, 19
Rose Medical, 117
RTSpect, 182

S

/s/, 29, **149**
Sacks, Stephen, 93, 117
SAILS app, 45, 56, 74
Same–different pairs, for perceptual therapy, 74–75, **75**
SATPAC. *See* Systematic Articulation Training Program Accessing Computers
Secord, Wayne, 114
SeeMore Imaging, 194
Self-assessment, 91
Self-generated stimuli, 92
Self-monitoring, 91–92, 110–111, 122–123
Sensory awareness, 120
Silent otitis, 74
Single sound errors, 6
Singleton, /r/ mastery as, 35, **36–37**, 57
Skelton, Steven, 130
SmartPalate system, 165
SMC. *See* Speech motor chaining
Sona-Speech II system, 182
Sound approximation, 117
Sound shaping, 117
Sounds of Speech, 117, 156
Spectrograms
    description of, viii, 13
    as visual acoustic feedback, 173, **174**, 177
Speech
    as complex motor task, 79
    flexibility in, 79
    internal feedback during, 144–145
    physiology of, 13
    tactile feedback in, 145–147
    visual input in acquisition of, 155–156

Speech Assessment and Interactive Learning System. *See* SAILS app
Speech Buddies, 121, 148–153, **149**, **151–152**, 154, 169, 197, **198**
Speech Correction (Van Riper), 102
Speech motor chaining, 81, 87, 90, 92
Speech perception
    description of, 4
    motor theory of, 5
    /r/ error as problem of, 45–47
Speech production errors, 46
Speech Production–Perception Task, 55–56, 63–67, 74
Speech services
    academic underperformance as qualification for, 7
    Individuals with Disabilities Education Act criteria for, 7
Speech sound(s)
    contextual influences on, 29
    gender differences in, 21–22
    mastery of, 34–35
    requirements for production of, 47
Speech sound disorders
    in children, 120
    tactile sensitivity in, 145–146
Speech sound errors
    articulation rates affected by, 52
    bullying because of, 6
    hearing screening for, 50
    in K–3 students, 1
    oromyofunctional disorders and, 53
    as perceptual problems, 4, 54–56
    as phonological problems, 56–57
    in pre-K students, 1
    prevalence of, 1
    in 7–12 grade students, 1
    speech perception difficulties with, 46
    study methods for
        acoustic analysis, 13
        electromagnetic articulography, 14
        magnetic resonance imaging, 13
        palatography. *See* Palatography
        ultrasound, 11–13, **12**
        x-rays, 11
    tongue thrust and, 53

Speech sound errors *(continued)*
vocal tract narrowing for production
of, 3
Speech sound interventions
discrimination training in, 45
goal of, 76
phonological therapy, 76–78
SP-PT. *See* Speech Production–
Perception Task
staRT, 182
State dependent learning, 90
Static palatography, 9
Stimulability
assessment of, 53–54, 61–62
probe, 61–62, 139
role of, 50
Stop consonants, 114
Systematic Articulation Training
Program Accessing Computers
advantages of, 139, **198**
description of, 115, 136–138, 197
disadvantages of, **198**
Establishment phase, 137
evidence for, 138–139, **140**
Generalization/Transfer phase, 138
nonsense words in, **137**
Practice phase, 137–138
r elicitation using, 125–126
studies of, 121, 138–139, **140**
tongue depressors used as bite-
block in, 121, **122**, 147

T

Tactile feedback
description of, 143
/r/ and, 145
removable intraoral appliance for,
153–154
in speech, 145–147
Speech Buddies, 121, 148–153, **149**,
151–152, 154, 197, **198**
supplemental input, 147–148
Tactile sensitivity, 145–147
Teeth, 52
Third formant, 21
Tongue
bracing of, 26–27, **28**, 116, 127
growth patterns of, 52

in /r/ production, 3, 20, 22–26, **25**
ultrasound of, **12**, 21, 188–189, **189**
vocal tract contact with, 26–27, **28**,
145
Tongue blades, 147
Tongue depressors, **122**, 147, 154
Tongue root, 4, 127
Tongue shapes
alternative tongue tip rhotic, 23
in British English, 22
bunched, 20, 23–26, **25**, **84**, 116–117
bunched rhotic, 23
contextual differences in, 28–29, **29**
retroflex, 3, 20, 23–26, **25**, **84**, 117
x-ray studies, 22
Tongue thrust, 53
Tongue-tie, 51
Tonsil enlargement, 51
Touch cues, 118
Traditional articulation therapy
advantages of, **198**
bottom-up approach, 129–130
concurrent treatment, 129–136,
134–135, 139, **198**
dimensions of, 102
disadvantages of, **198**
ear training, 105–106, 108
evidence to support, 108–112, **113**
homework in, 93–94, 111
modifications in, 123
nonsense material, 106
/r/ elicitation, 114–119
randomized treatment sequence in,
130, **131–132**
reconfiguration, 107
self-monitoring in, 110–111,
122–123
summary of, **112**
treatment hierarchy, 129
treatment sequence, 102, **103–104**,
112, **113**, 123
Van Riper's approach, 102, 104–110,
122–123
visual input and, 156

U

Ultrasound
accessibility issues, 197

advantages of, 186, 195, **198**
constriction studies using, 21
costs of, 190–191
disadvantages of, 186, 195, **198**
equipment for, 194–195
frequencies used by, 187
image capture with, 188
principles of, 12, 185–187
/r/ error applications of, 185–186,
    194
real-time nature of, 186
safety of, 191
speech remediation uses of
    advantages of, 185–186, 195
    clinician training and orientation
        for, 190
    equipment for, 194–195
    evidence for, 194
    procedure for, **188–189**, 188–190
    safety concerns, 191
speech studies using, 11–13, **12**
tongue bracing studies using, 27
tongue imaging using, **12**, 21,
    188–189, **189**
transducers, 187
visual feedback via
    basics of, 187–194
    description of, 171, 187
    establishment and stabilization
        with, 192–194, **193**
    orientation to, 191–192, **192**
University of Iowa Research
    Foundation, 117

V

Van Riper, Charles, 102, 104–110,
    122–123
Velars, 114
Verbal feedback, 143–144
Visible Speech, 13
Visi-Pitch system, 182
Visual acoustic feedback
    abstract nature of, 169, 171
    advantages of, 169, 182–183, **198**
    attentional focus of, 171
    basics of, 175, 177–179
    characteristics of, 171–172
    disadvantages of, 183, **198**

equipment for, 182
establishment and stabilization with,
    178–179
evidence for, 179, **180–181**
linear predictive coding spectrum
    displays, 173, 175, **176**
orientation to, 177, **178**
overview of, 169–170
/r/ errors treated with, 179,
    180–181
/r/ information, 172
spectrograms, 173, **174**, 177
speech movements, 169
studies of, 179, **180–181**
types of, 172–175
unique nature of, 171–172
Visual feedback
    acoustic. *See* Visual acoustic
        feedback
    advantages of, 156–157
    age limitations for, 199
    challenges of providing, 157
    description of, 94, 117
    electropalatography as. *See*
        Electropalatography
    ultrasound as. *See* Ultrasound, visual
        feedback via
Visual input
    mirrors for, 156
    in speech acquisition, 155–156
    traditional therapy and, 156
Vocal tract
    gender differences in, 5, 21
    narrowing of, for /r/ production, 3,
        26
    tongue contact with, 26–27, **28**, 145
Vowel, /r/ as, 14, **15**
Vygotsky's zone of proximal
    development, 88

W

[w] substitution for /r/
    description of, vii, 3, 43–44
    as gliding, 48
    /r/ distortion versus, 44–45, 47
    stimulability of, 50
WASP, 182
Watch-and-see approach, 40

wavesurfer.js, 182
Whole-language intervention, ix

X

X-ray(s)
    speech studies using, 11

tongue bracing studies using, 27,
    28
X-ray microbeam, 11

Z

Zone of proximal development, 88